Ketogenic Diet for Beginners

Over 60 instant pot recipes and a 14-day Keto diet meal plan for weight loss and healthy living

ISBN-13: 978-1721656912
ISBN-10: 172165691X

Text Copyright © Hanna Soloha

Legal & Disclaimer

The information contained in this book and its contents is not designed to replace or take the place of any form of medical or professional advice; and is not meant to replace the need for independent medical, financial, legal or other professional advice or services, as may be required. The content and information in this book have been provided for educational and entertainment purposes only.

The content and information contained in this book have been compiled from sources deemed reliable, and it is accurate to the best of the Author's knowledge, information, and belief. However, the Author cannot guarantee its accuracy and validity and cannot be held liable for any errors and/or omissions. Further, changes are periodically made to this book as and when needed. Where appropriate and/or necessary, you must consult a professional (including but not limited to your doctor, attorney, financial advisor or such other professional advisor) before using any of the suggested remedies, techniques, or information in this book.

Upon using the contents and information contained in this book, you agree to hold harmless the Author from and against any damages, costs, and expenses, including any legal fees potentially resulting from the application of any of the information provided by this book. This disclaimer applies to any loss, damages or injury caused by the use and application, whether directly or indirectly, of any advice or information presented, whether for breach of contract, tort, negligence, personal injury, criminal intent, or under any other cause of action. You agree to accept all risks of using the information presented in this book.

You agree that by continuing to read this book, where appropriate and/or necessary, you shall consult a professional (including but not limited to your doctor, attorney, or financial advisor or such other advisor as needed) before using any of the suggested remedies, techniques, or information in this book.

Introduction

We all have wishes in life. Our daily lives and activities are driven and inspired by our much cherished goals. All I've wished for in life is to always be a problem-solver to life's numerous challenges. As a foodie, I decided to contribute my quota to writing a ketogenic diet cookbook. This cookbook is informative and offers rich and amazing recipes for your reading and dining pleasure.

You deserve the best. When reading this e-book not only will you learn how to prepare each meal but I will also provide a two-week meal plan that will serve as an invaluable guide for you.

Make this book your best kitchen companion! *You will lose weight without losing value* and be healthy always!

Chapter 1: What is a ketogenic diet?

The basics of ketogenic diet

Before getting started, **I want to tell you what motivated me into putting this piece** together. *Out of love for money?* No! In fact, writing a book for monetary gains doesn't get one very far. What is the essence of living a displeasing life just because you are out of shape? Why should you be denied living an active life and enjoying a social life? This book was borne out of this concern and provides not only a feasible solution, but a practical and economical one. Something that can be adopted as a lifestyle!

The major aim of a ketogenic diet is to put the body on a metabolic path referred to as "ketosis". This is accomplished through adopting a low carbohydrate diet that is high in fat. On a ketogenic diet the body does not depend on sugar for energy production. Instead, the body relies on fat for energy. *Does that sound strange?* Well, it isn't conventional but full of goodies! Keep reading to discover the *abnormal normalcy.*

Ketosis is the process of producing ketones with fat in the liver. This bodily process is naturally initiated to keep us fueled with energy even with reduced food consumption. That is why the formula for a ketogenic diet is always high fats (75%) + low carbohydrates (5%) + moderate protein (20%) = healthy diet.

This chart illustrates the ketogenic diet formula:

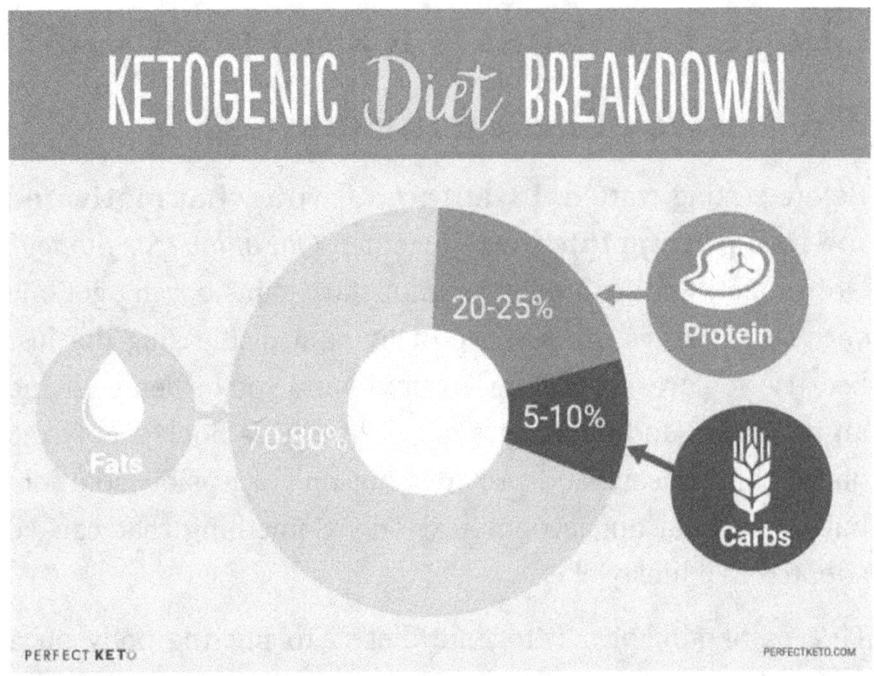

The sole aim of every disciplined keto-adapted person is to compel the body into the state of ketosis by starving carbohydrates instead of calories.

The natural process of energy production in the body

Adenosine Triphosphate (ATP) is the only energy source to all human cells. The ATP derives energy from fats, carbohydrates and proteins. However, just a small dimension of the ATP is stored for human metabolism. Thus, there are three natural ways energy production occurs in the human body:

The first form of energy production is through aerobic phosphorylation. Here, cells burn glucose with the use of oxygen to produce the ATP. The energy produced through this means is used in performing daily routines, physical exercises and embarking on long distance treks. However, the aerobic respiration is a weak energy source.

The second form of energy production is anaerobic glycolysis or respiration. This takes place in cytoplasm. This energy is most useful for short duration exercises that don't last for more than 3 minutes and sprints. It is partially burning glucose without oxygen to produce ATP.

The last production method is through ATP Phosphocreatine (ATP-PT) which is reputed as being the fastest energy source. Whenever the body is in rapid need of energy, it taps all the cells in small quantity. However, this energy burns at an inexplicably fast rate. This type of energy, which doesn't involve the use of oxygen, is used in power or weight lifting scenarios.

All these processes are the natural ways in which energy is produced in the body.

Change in the natural process of the body with a ketogenic diet

An indispensable effect of a ketogenic diet is that it changes some of the natural processes of the body. Once you're keto-adapted, your body's energy is not solely tied to glucose as an energy source. It shifts to fats produced with a substance called ketone in the liver. Once the ketones find their way into your blood, the body switches over and the body cells derive power through the ketones for daily activities. The incredibility of changing the body's process from over-reliance on glucose to moderate amounts of ketones for healthy living is the major selling point for the ketogenic diet.

Take a look at the chart below to see how it works:

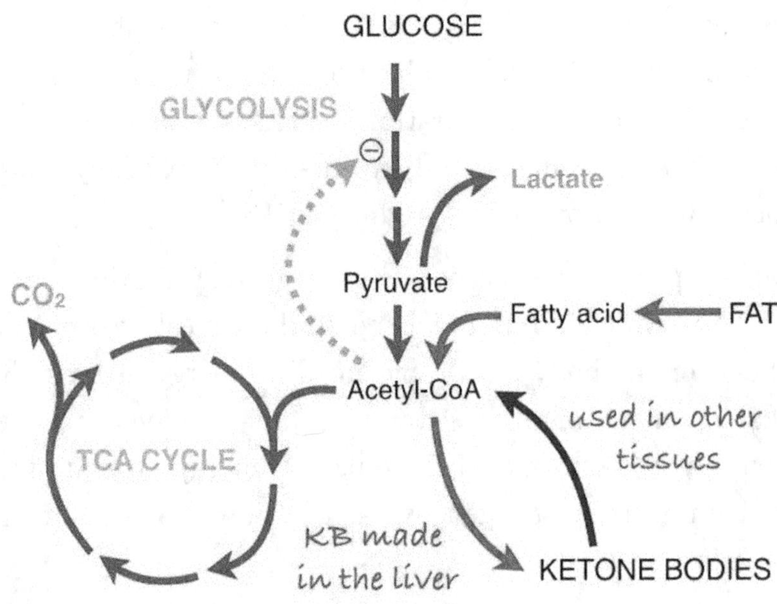

What happens to your body when on a ketogenic diet?

Going on a ketogenic diet is a lofty idea. It is good for you to know how your body functions and what to expect when you're on a ketogenic diet so as to get the most benefits.

During the adjustment period when your body switches gears on energy sources, there is a likelihood of fatigue, brain fog and sometimes bad breath. These issues will subside on their own once you've fully adjusted to your new lifestyle.

Weight loss is another common occurrence. Research studies have confirmed that much of the weight loss that occurs during the initial stage of going keto is water weight and as such can be regained within a short period of time. Also, the hormones are expected to circulate and they can promote the storage of fats.

In addition, since there is a reduction in your intake of carbohydrates, this also reduces the volume of fiber you consume and may lead to constipation. For the beginners who are just consuming large quantity of fats for the first time, diarrhea is another common occurrence. Again, it takes just a short adjustment period for all these symptoms to subside on their own. To be on the safe side, the amount of carbohydrates you consume should be rich in fiber to prevent constipation.

What is ketosis?

I have discussed a part of this concept while discussing the basics of a ketogenic diet. Ketosis is a metabolic state whereby the body produces ketones with fats in the liver as a source of energy in the absence of glucose.

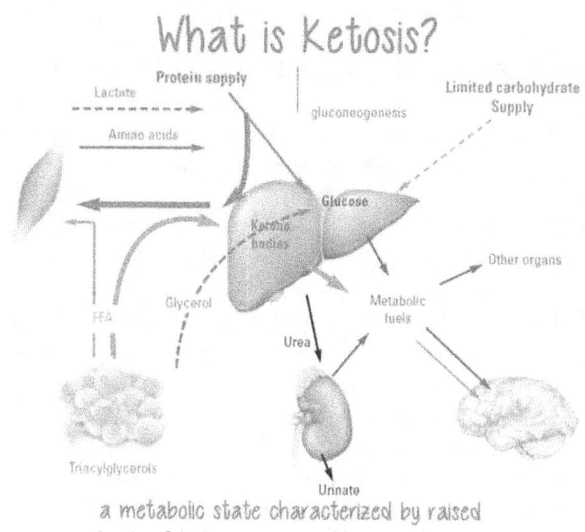

Credit: Siim land

Once the shift to the intake of a high-fat diet with low carbs happens, metabolism occurs through the burning of fats for energy instead of from carbohydrate contents.

How does ketosis improve health?

There are many studies that outline how beneficial ketosis is to your health. In fact, many of the researchers are of the opinion that being on a keto diet is the best decision one can make in life.

I know you'll be a doubting Thomas about this until you try it out. Seeing is believing!

Ketosis reduces your appetite. This is an advantage that this diet has over many others that have forced people out of them. Ketones do not need high amounts of calories to function effectively.

In addition, ketosis ensures that the fats in your body are not concentrated in one place but are properly circulated to ensure weight loss. Those struggling with obesity will find this point good news.

PerfectKeto in this chart illustrates this health benefit:

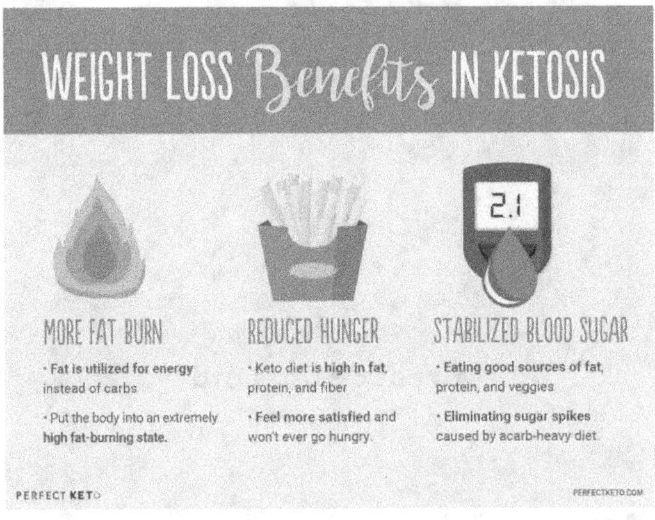

More importantly, ketosis prevents fatty liver diseases. Ketosis takes place in the liver and instead of leaving the fats in the liver without any use, it burns them as a source of energy for the body.

Why should you give up on carbohydrates?

Are you still adamant about consuming high carbs? There are many untold benefits to giving up carbohydrates:

Instead of your body relying on sugar as its energy source, it will be compelled to switch over to burning fats. Notably, fats are already stored in the body and are easily accessible.

Given that ketosis reduces hunger, a keto diet can make travel simpler. Some people cannot travel due to their poor eating habits. *My apology for the bombshell but it's just the naked truth that must be embraced.* Unfortunately, calories don't satiate hunger; instead you should consume more nutrient-based diets like keto. When you're on a keto diet, you feel less hungry and there is less of a need for constant snacking.

Also, when you give up carbohydrates, you reduce your risk of diabetes. Most carbohydrates have high sugar content and when you consume them incessantly, they have both short and long term health effects such as diabetes, which is commonly caused by high sugar intake. Is this convincing enough for you to call it a day with carbohydrates?

In the same vein, when you reduce your intake of high carbs, you become more strengthened. Many other diets don't have proteins that will build your muscles and strengthen you. When you switch over from high simple carbs to a keto diet, the source of energy for your body becomes steady and reliable. Thus, your body doesn't have to rely on a high intake of calories all the time.

Below is a table of the grams of carbohydrates you consume in common cereals, cakes, desserts and biscuits:

Cereals, biscuits and desserts	Amount of carbohydrate (g)	Kcal
Boiled pearl barley	-	28
Chocolate biscuit	20	67
Rye crisp bread	20	70
Ginger nut	15	79
Semi-sweet gingernut	15	75
Short-sweet gingernut	15	62
Bran wheat	8	27
Brown sliced bread	25	48
Lebanese pita	¼ -25	53
Sliced wholemeal	25	47
Brown roll	35	57
Fruit cake	60	58
Sponge cake	60	53
Cheesecake	120	35
Cornflakes	30	87
Crumpet	50	52
Custard	70	4

Doughnut	40	49
Full-fat soya	-	24
Low-fat soya	-	28
Fruit pie	150	57
Lemon meringue pie	120	46
Pancake	75	36
Muesli	30	56
Boiled spaghetti	120	26
Flaky pastry	-	41
Boiled rice	160	30
Wheat	35	75
Dried yeast	-	4

Courtesy: apjc.nhri.org

Going keto for beginners

Truthfully, it can be difficult to go keto, especially when the people around you are not supportive and encouraging. You might have a spouse or friend who is consuming the high sugar diet that you were used to right in front of you. ***But despite these temptations, be strong in keto and its ways!*** The plain truth is that you can always survive if you're serious and focused in your newly adopted lifestyle. Before going keto, you were used to the intake of a high-carb diet that supplied your body energy through blood glucose. The blood glucose increases the level of insulin which negatively enhances the storage of fat in the body.

However, keto as a low-carb diet rich in fat brings about a state of metabolism known as ketosis. Instead of glycolysis, ketosis burns the body fat for energy through a normal process. It burns the fat reserve when your body system is low on carbs.

As a beginner, a concern might be how the parts of the body that solely need glucose as fuel will work effectively. The answer to this is simple: there is an adequate amount of glycerol that can be obtained through dietary fats, which the body rapidly converts to glucose through gluconeogenesis.

As a beginner, one of the best ways of embracing this diet is to consume a keto diet at least 6 times in a week. After you're fully *keto-adapted*, there would be a rapid decrease of glycogen in your body. An untold advantage of this is that it increases your energy level and reduces your weight. So if you still yield to the "temptation of the world" and stop eating a keto diet, it will be easy for you to return to keto eating compared to when you first started. Isn't this good news worth celebrating? *Yes, celebrate with a keto diet!*

Is Ketosis dangerous?

One of the major misconceptions about nutritional ketosis is that it has been mistaken for diabetic ketoacidosis (DKA) by some medical experts and as such considered a life-threatening condition. This is far from the truth. ***Never listen to the echoes of the 'confusionists'.***

DKA is a sudden drop in the insulin level in the body. Even with the high presence of glucose, a diabetic patient cannot function without insulin. Problems arise with a diabetic patient as they cannot produce insulin and can't continuously produce ketones. So, when the ketone level increases beyond the normal level, it results in a pH imbalance in the patient, leading to critical illness.

The good news is that this condition can never occur in a person who manages to produce small amounts of insulin. Fortunately, a keto-adapted person maintains a balanced pH level between 0.5 to 3.0 mM, which does not fall within the 'harm range'. Thus, nutritional ketosis is not synonymous with diabetic ketoacidosis.

The brain needs both glucose and ketones to function optimally. While the body can only store glucose for one day, it relies on ketones induced by the liver through amino acids to keep functioning. If not, it will lead to hypoglycemia, a condition that can be fatal. Hence, ketones become an indispensable part of our well-being.

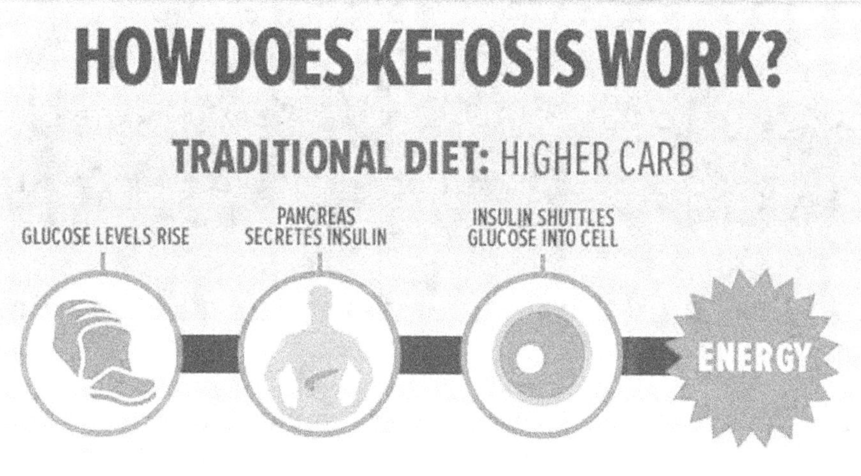

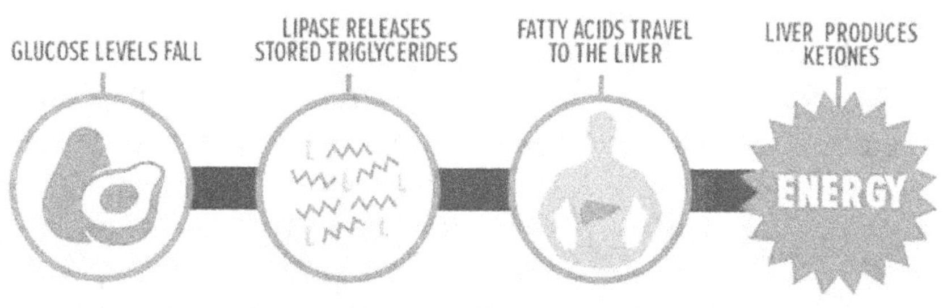

Credit: Human Rebuild

Notably, it is advisable that diabetic patients consult with their personal doctors before going keto. This is more specific for type 1 diabetic patients whose diet may need to be modified when consuming low-carb diets.

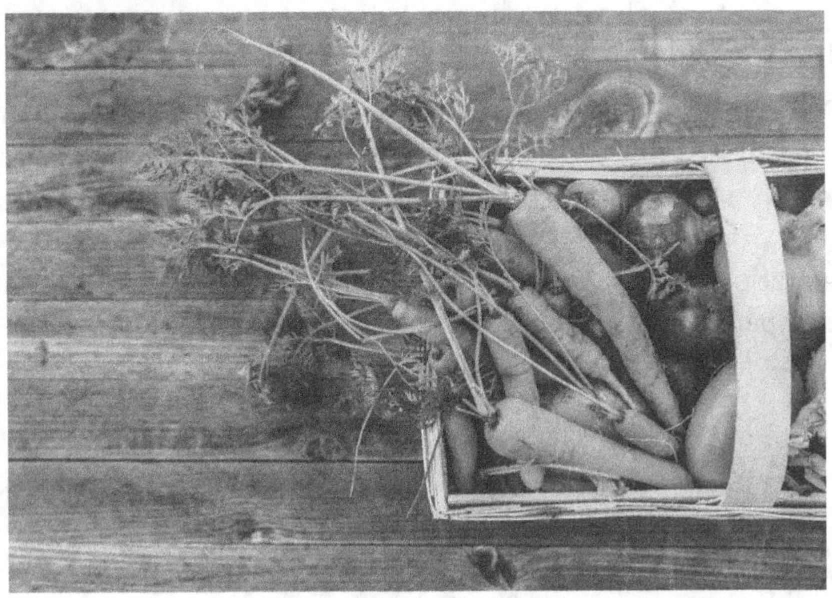

Do I need medical supervision for a ketogenic diet?

You don't necessarily need medical supervision while going keto if you're not suffering from any form of diabetes. However, there are some precautions you need to take in order to get the best out of this master-class diet.

First, please go through medical screening to ascertain whether you are free to be *keto-adapted*. There may be an undetected health condition that might warrant that you eat more carbohydrates. Please note, pregnant women should not adopt this diet. Additionally, if you're recovering from an eating disorder, this diet may not be best for you; *you're in a reserve mode until you fully recuperate.*

Consulting your doctor before going on this diet is the best way to stay safe and avoid potential complications. Your doctor will be able to advise you on the best diet for you.

Apart from this, all you need is an occasional keto test to know if you're still on the right track or if you need to adjust. This will also help you to know if you're getting the desired results you want.

Chapter 2: The Benefits of a Ketogenic Diet

Now that you understand the concepts underlying a ketogenic diet, let's discuss the advantages of this healthy and researched-acknowledged diet. No doubt, the advantages of this diet have been its major selling point over other diets. Seven major benefits of a ketogenic diet are discussed in this *cookbook to further bolster your faith in the keto journey:*

Decrease of appetite/ lack of hunger

Don't be deceived; calories don't satisfy you. They only encourage continuous unhealthy intake of sugar. What brings satisfaction are healthy fats and moderate proportions of proteins and low carbs. This is the formula for a ketogenic diet. So, once you eat your meals and you're committed to your diet, your level of hunger will decrease. A keto diet kills undue longing for snacks and other unhealthy foods. This diet has been proven to have the ability to normalize the hunger hormone known as Ghrelin. With this diet, your refrigerator and pantry can stay full as you will no longer have undue zeal for unhealthy foods.

More importantly, positive changes in hunger level can lead to sustainable and permanently weight loss. According to studies, those who lose weight while on keto don't regain weight when they return to their usual nutrition. Also, keto diet preserves the normal calorie level and the amount of food intake.

Absence of jumps in blood sugar

A natural way to lower your blood sugar is through a ketogenic diet, according to studies. Foods high in carbohydrates shoot up your blood sugar which is very harmful to your body. People are constantly being deceived by the mediation role of insulin. But the truth is once the sugar content becomes too high in the body, insulin becomes incapacitated and this leads to many problems.

The best assistance you can render to your body is to switch over to a ketogenic diet that naturally lowers blood sugar levels before it gets out of hand. When you become keto-adapted, your body's focus shifts from glucose and other sugar-related contents to fats. Keto foods like blueberries, turmeric, cabbage and lemons help reduce blood sugar level.

Low blood pressure

Another huge benefit of a keto diet to a disciplined *keto-er* is that is lowers blood pressure level. High blood pressure is an open gate to many other rampant diseases such as stroke, kidney infection, heart failure, among others. Studies show that when you consume food very low in carbohydrates, you reduce the chances of raising your blood pressure level. These diseases thrive on sugar. Once they are deprived of this, they become extremely weak and unable to attack the protective cells.

In research carried out by **Healthline**, it was discovered that a keto diet can effectively lower blood pressure within a few months of its administration.

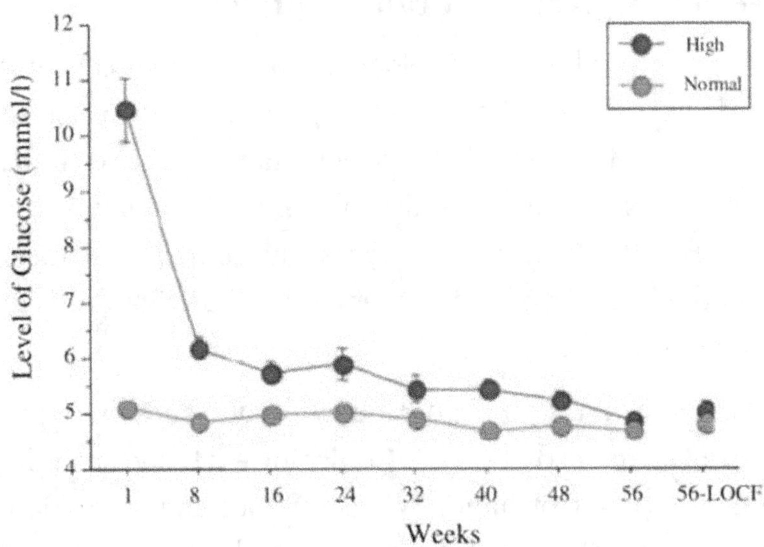

Fig. 6 Changes in the level of blood glucose after the administration of ketogenic diet for 56 weeks

Courtesy: healthline.com

Elevated HDL Levels

HDL is commonly referred to as the *good cholesterol*. Instead of carrying cholesterol around the body like LDL, the HDL moves it directly to the liver where it can be processed and used positively before being excreted out of the body.

Research-backed claims show that the best way to increase the HDL is through the consumption of fats, a major nutrient of a ketogenic diet. A major benefit of increased HDL is lowered risk of heart disease. Thus, a ketogenic diet helps prevent heart diseases.

Increased weight loss

Increased weight loss is the most obvious benefit of a ketogenic diet. Some may think this benefit is overstated, but it is just the irresistibly obvious point! Simple carbs make you gain unnecessary weight. If you desire weight loss through nutrition, the best option available for you is to go keto.

According to studies, people on low-carb diets like keto lose weight at a desired level and pace compared to those who pursue low-fat diets. You don't need to starve yourself to lose weight. Most keto recipes can be prepared in less than 30 minutes. And in this book, thanks to instant pot for its multiple functions, you will learn several keto recipes that can be prepared quickly! Keto is simply the awaiting miracle for your weight loss.

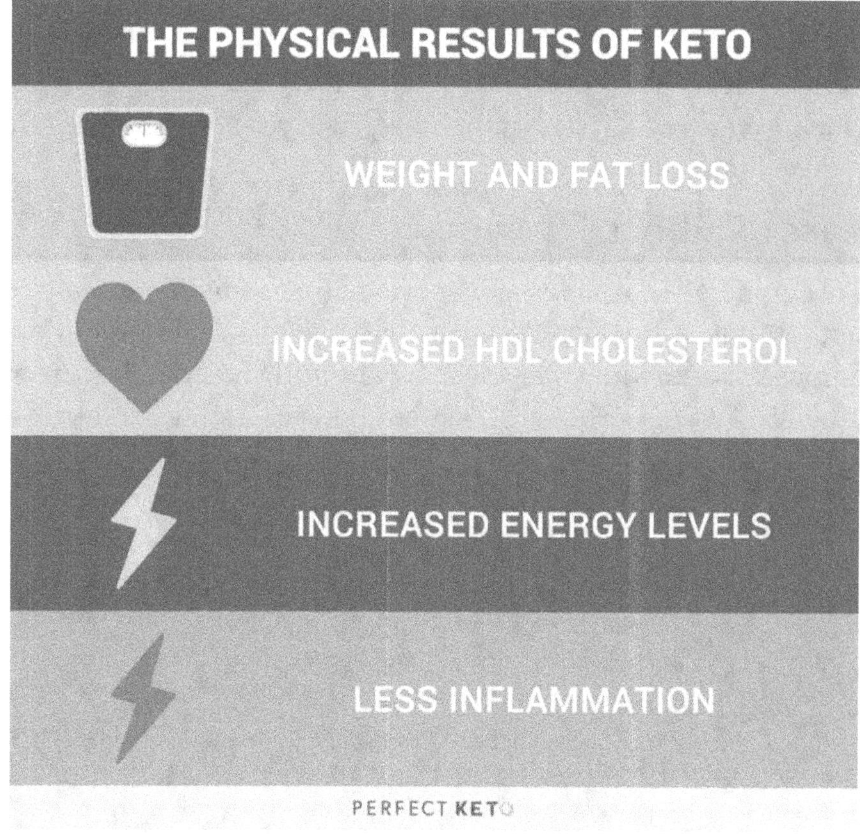

If you want to succeed in long-term weight loss, you need to be disciplined in being *keto-adapted* so as not to regain weight; ***make keto a lifestyle and not just a diet!***

Strict avoidance of carbohydrates is the key to being fully keto-adapted. Keto requires a capital NO to carbs; even a slice of banana will break the chain of the mechanism. Once you consume carbohydrates, the brain is quickly alerted to the intake of glucose and instantly, the ketosis process stops.

Reduced triglycerides

This is the last benefit I will discuss in this delectable book. Triglycerides are described as fat molecules. Triglycerides, when they gain full access into the blood pose a great threat to the heart. However, the major means of these molecules being driven into the blood are carbohydrates. Triglycerides thrive on fructose, an end product of simple carbs.

Once you're on a ketogenic diet, triglycerides are greatly reduced in your body.

Loss of adipose tissue

This point is for athletes and sportsmen in general. Yes, you're not left out in this healthy diet. Keto ensures rapid loss of the adipose tissue while the muscles are still intact. Apart from athletes, all those who desire a tight body can always bank on a keto diet.

Chapter 3: Recommendations for feeding a ketogenic diet

Now, let's dip into the cookbook and I urge you to pay close attention to every detail discussed herein. Adopting the new lifestyle a ketogenic diet provides must be guided by instructions.

There are recommendations for eating a ketogenic diet that provide greater results.

Proteins

One of the major shortcomings of newbies going keto is consuming an inappropriate amount of proteins. Apart from reducing the rate of carbs in your diet, the quantity of proteins must also be moderate.

A high intake of protein is bad because your major intent of going keto is to switch the body over from using glucose as a means of energy production to using fats. However, if you eat too much protein, the body will manipulate its building block (amino acids) to produce glucose (what you were actually running away from).

Now that you've been told about the evil of consuming a high amount of protein, the question is, how then do we know the right quantity of protein to add to a keto diet? Read on!

Diligence and observance! Usually, the amount of protein you need in your diet is between 20 to 25%. For a beginner, always use the <u>keto app</u> to track the exact quantity of protein you need at a given time.

Given that you're advised to eat a moderate amount of protein, ensure that they are topnotch and healthy. The best sources of protein are bison, beef, lamb, sardines, tuna, liver meats and salmon. Please, **NEVER** eat processed food as protein because they usually contain sugar; go for natural sources always.

Fats and oil

This food group should be the core of what you consume. Generally, fat should amount to 70-80% of your ketogenic diet. Your fats should always be from natural and pure sources such as nuts and meats. In addition, fat supplements with a lot of monounsaturated fats should be your best choice. Some of these supplements are olive oil, butter, coconut oil, macadamia, avocado, lard, ghee and others.

Since fats contribute to a large chunk of your daily diet, choose fats that are high quality and easy to sustain access to so as not to be easily frustrated. In addition, you can be dynamic about it and vary your fat sources. Don't indulge in the consumption of unhealthy fats so as to avoid exposing your body to threats.

Vegetables and fruits

Vegetables and fruits are an indispensable part of a ketogenic diet. You need to exercise caution when choosing veggies to consume. Those that are unhealthy that have a high rate of carbs should be weeded out of your list or reduced to the barest minimum.

Ideally, the vegetables you should consume while on keto should be rich in nutrients with an inconsequential amount of carbohydrates. Cruciferous veggies should be your major target. This includes leafy and dark vegetables. Whether frozen or fresh, ensure the vegetables you're consuming are nutritious and healthy.

Examples of fruits and vegetables that should be added to your meals are green beans, blackberries, green bell pepper, cabbage, spinach, raspberries, baby bella mushrooms and broccoli.

The table below will guide the choice of fruits and veggies you consume:

Veggies and Fruits	Amount of carbohydrates (g)	Kcal
Apple	100	9
Apricots	3-100	6
Canned apricots	100	28
Banana	100	19
Blackberries	100	6
Cherries	20-100	10
Black currants	90	7
Canned fruit salad	120	25
Black grapes	20-100	13
White grapes	20-100	15
Canned juice	120	8
Canned guavas	100	18
Lemon slices	2-15	3
Juice	15	2
Loganberries	100	3
Mango	100	15
Canned mango	100	20
Fresh juice	120	9
Pawpaw	100	11
Canned pawpaw	100	17

Whole passion fruit	30	3
Mandarins	2-100	11
Prunes	8-80	34
Raw quince	100	6
Dried raisins	20	64
Raspberries	100	6
Canned raspberries	100	23
Raspberries, stewed, no-sugar	100	6
Strawberries	10-100	6
Canned strawberries	100	21
Dried sultanas	15	65
Watermelon	260	3
Pineapple	80	12
Peach	120	8
Whole grapefruit	200	3
Avocado pear	½ -50	2

Courtesy: apjcn.nhri.org

NOTE: The amount of carbohydrates in each item is in grams (g).

Dairy

The consumption of dairy is dependent on the meal at hand. While keeping your dairy consumption at a very moderate level, ensure that you always consume products that are organic and raw. For your keto diet, always select dairy products with high-fat ratio over low-fat options. This will bolster your health and will contribute to fat burning for energy.

Examples of keto-based dairy products are whipping cream, hard cheeses such as feta, swiss, parmesan, etc; Greek yogurt; soft cheeses such as colby, blue, brie, mozzarella, etc; other examples are cream cheese, cottage cheese, crème fraiche, etc.

Although dairy products are great sources for accumulating the right fats in the body, let it always ring at the back of your mind that they have some contents of proteins in them and as such, should be consumed moderately, especially when pairing them with meals dominated by proteins.

Nuts and seeds

The best nuts and seeds for a keto diet are roasted ones that are rich in nutrients. Peanuts are not part of keto diet foods. You may always add nuts as a means of texture to your meals. While others eat them as snacks, it is pertinent to reiterate that this can have a negative effect on those who want to lose weight with a keto diet.

Even though nuts are wonderful fat sources, they also contain some carbohydrates and proteins. This is why you need to limit the amount of nuts you consume. Examples of nuts to be adapted into your keto diets are pecans, brazil nuts, almonds, macadamia nuts and hazelnuts.

Spices and additives

When it comes to choosing sauces and seasoning, you need to be on alert more than ever before. They can be enemies of your diet. So many seasonings contain sugar that will be processed to glucose when eaten. There are just a few reliable ones on the market.

Also, spices contain some amounts of carbohydrates, so they must be added to your meals with moderation. Examples of spices that can be added to your keto diet are basil, parsley, thyme, rosemary, chili powder, cayenne pepper, cumin and oregano.

What to drink

A common issue for ketogenic diet beginners is hydration, especially those prone to bladder issues and other urinary disorders. It is best that you drink at least 3 liters of water a day; you need water to survive and should not trade it for anything. Ketoproof coffee is an option but it is not a better alternative to water. Flavored beverages should not exceed 2 cups in your daily diet.

Apart from water, other beverages to drink are coffee, tea, almond milk, broth, hard liquor, diet soda and flavoring.

What should be avoided

Now that we've discussed recommendations for eating a ketogenic diet, let's discuss the things that should be avoided when you go keto. In order to be on the safe side, **stick to all the foods I've recommended to you at the appropriate quantity.**

Here are five major items you should always run away from once you are on keto:

Sugar. This is a no-gray-area for you. Chocolate bars, sweets, candy, juice, frozen treats and breakfast cereals should be avoided.

Starch. Once you're on a ketogenic diet, every form of starchy foods such as bread, sweet potatoes, pasta, potato chips, french fries, porridge and others in the same category should be avoided. Strike them off your dietary list.

WHAT FOODS TO:

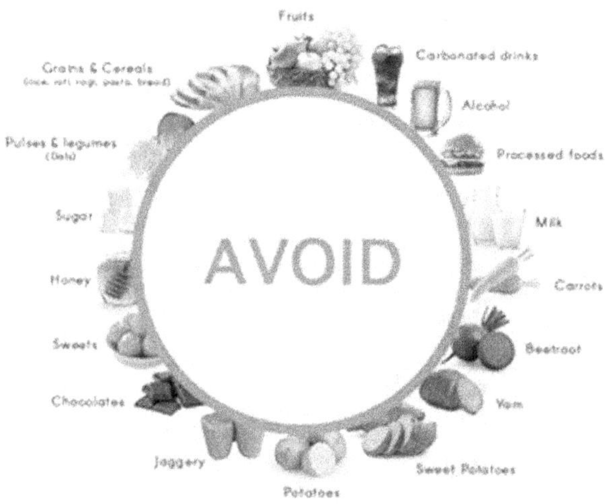

Credit: Gympik

Beer. This liquid bread has a high amount of carbs. They aren't helpful to your new lifestyle.

Fruits. Many fruits are sugary with a high content of carbs. This becomes more dangerous when they're processed.

Margarine. This is filled with high artificial omega 6 fat. Apart from its bad taste, there are no health benefits linked to it. In fact, it has been medically linked as a potential cause of allergies, inflammatory diseases and asthma.

Chapter 4: Tips to help you succeed on a ketogenic diet

Truth be told, going keto is one of the difficult decisions one can make in life as it requires discipline and commitment. I'm going to share some invaluable tips on how to succeed on a ketogenic diet.

The diagram below is your *Ten Commandments* to follow if you plan to succeed on a ketogenic diet.

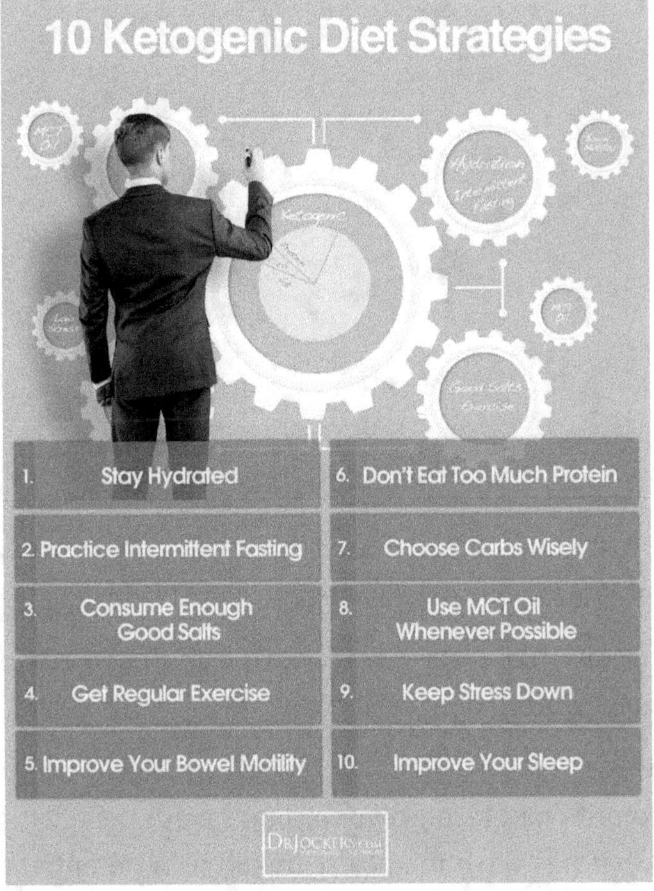

Calorie intake and ketogenic diet

If your primary purpose of going keto is to lose weight, you have no other option than to do away with the intake of calories for some period of time. You start what is technically referred to as intermittent fasting (IF). With intermittent fasting, you'll become keto-adapted faster.

During this period, the body quickly depletes the excess glucose in your body so as to allow you to go into ketosis. For beginners, I recommend fasting within a daily window. Apart from being the most popular IF method, it has proven to be the most result-oriented. Try skipping your breakfast and then consume food from noon until about 8pm.

Other forms of intermittent fasting are alternate day fasting, meal skipping and only eating while hungry.

Hydration and ketogenic diet

Staying hydrated is one of the difficulties that beginners on keto encounter. Always remember that you lose more water than you retain while on keto, so always drink a lot of water. Ideally, a minimum of 32 oz should be your morning 'dose' and another 48 oz of water at noon. Generally, you should aim for drinking about a gallon of water daily.

When you're committed to this religiously, you avoid dehydration. Drink more water in the summer and after intense exercise sessions.

Ketogenic diet and your budget

The good news about going keto is that even when you're on a budget, you'll still get to eat healthy meals.

Always buy in bulk and freeze. Foods can be bought in bulk and frozen. Meats can be frozen for as long as six months. Same goes for butter, veggies and berries. Once you have some cash available, go shopping and freeze what you buy to last you longer. Even on rainy days, you'll have dietary options.

Also, make Amazon your go-to marketplace. There are numerous sellers of the same product in the marketplace and you can always get a fair price after checking out all the sellers.

In order not to eat out on the run, always prepare meals ahead. Check your itinerary and be sure when you'll have hectic days when you might not have the chance to cook. You can have quick options at home. You can even make your own bone broth from the scraps of other meals. Bone broth can be very expensive to buy, but amazingly easy to make! You can also keep your bacon butter and use it at a later time.

In the same vein, never miss the season for berries and vegetables. Buy them during their season at a fair price and freeze.

Traveling with keto food

Always on the road? *No worries! I've got you covered with a whole lot of ideas!* There's no reason for rushing. Always eat and be full before embarking on your trip. There's no better place to feel relaxed and eat if not your home.

Self-discipline also comes into play here. You need to be assertive in resisting offers of high-carb snacks made by flight attendants. Instead, always travel with self-prepared low-carb snacks. Some common snacks to always travel with are babybel cheese, crudité with dip, peeled hard-boiled eggs with some salt, butter, nuts, parmesan cheese crisps and olive oil for vegetables and salads. Keep your goodies packed in a container so as to keep them accessible for you at all times.

Also, you can always send hunger away with a sip of coffee or tea.

Better still, intermittent fasting is another option. After eating breakfast, you might decide to skip lunch then have dinner after your arrival to your destination.

If you're the restaurant type, there are some foods such as bread, pasta, cookies and other high-carb contents that you should never order. Instead, ask for veggies and butter or olive oil to eat your salad. In addition to this, drink a lot of water to stay hydrated.

Choice of fast food and keto

While on a ketogenic diet, eating out can be dangerous. I've often been at a crossroads where I have many errands to run and it's noon, yet nothing has passed through my esophagus. In this situation, there's no better choice than to resort to fast food. Then, how do you balance that with your keto diet?

There are many fast food restaurants offering diverse sit-down options and keto fast foods. Anytime you find yourself in any of these restaurants, always order veggies, meats and cheese. If you're ordering salad, take time to read the ingredients as many of them are made with high-carb products. To be on a safe side, always get salads with dressing on the side.

Most times, fried foods like chicken wings and mozzarella sticks have a high ratio of carbohydrates, so always avoid them. Also, you need to be careful with condiments that come with dressings. More flexibly, you can always make a special request. Surely not everybody wants to do this but you can keep yourself safe by making specific requests that protect you from consuming high-carb foods.

If you're not sure of the ingredients, why not just skip it?

Chapter 5: Ketogenic 14-Day Meal Plan

Day 1

Breakfast: Casserole

Lunch: Pork and kraut

Dinner: Taco salad

Day 2

Breakfast: Keto egg cups

Lunch: Shredded chicken

Dinner: Easy balsamic beef

Day 3

Breakfast: Hard boiled eggs

Lunch: Bruschetta chicken with zoodles

Dinner: Mississippi pot roast

Day 4

Breakfast: Eggs made five ways

Lunch: spareribs

Dinner: Citrus herb chicken chorizo

Day 5

Breakfast: Avocado with egg and fat bomb

Lunch: Bacon hash

Dinner: Meatballs and sauce

Day 6

Breakfast: No noodle lasagna

Lunch: Cobb salad

Dinner: Green beans casserole

Day 7

Breakfast: Keto poblano cheese quiche

Lunch: Crack chicken

Dinner: Creamed spinach

Day 8

Breakfast: Coconut porridge

Lunch: Chicken foot broth

Dinner: Shepherd's pie

Day 9

Breakfast: Dairy-free coconut yogurt

Lunch: Mustard, tarragon and chicken soup

Dinner: Parmesan

Day 10

Breakfast: Bacon and egg muffins

Lunch: Cauliflower soufflé

Dinner: Garlic butter chicken

Day 11

Breakfast: Ground beef omelet

Lunch: Arroz con pollo

Dinner: Coconut curry powder

Day 12

Breakfast: Philly cheese steak wraps

Lunch: Chinese chicken and broccoli

Dinner: Creamy chicken bacon chowder

Day 13

Breakfast: Broccoli ham and pepper frittata

Lunch: Mexican-style pork shoulders tacos

Dinner: Butter chicken curry

Day 14

Breakfast: Pumpkin pie pudding

Lunch: Shredded chicken

Dinner: Smothered pork chops

Ketogenic Breakfast

Keto Egg Cups on the run

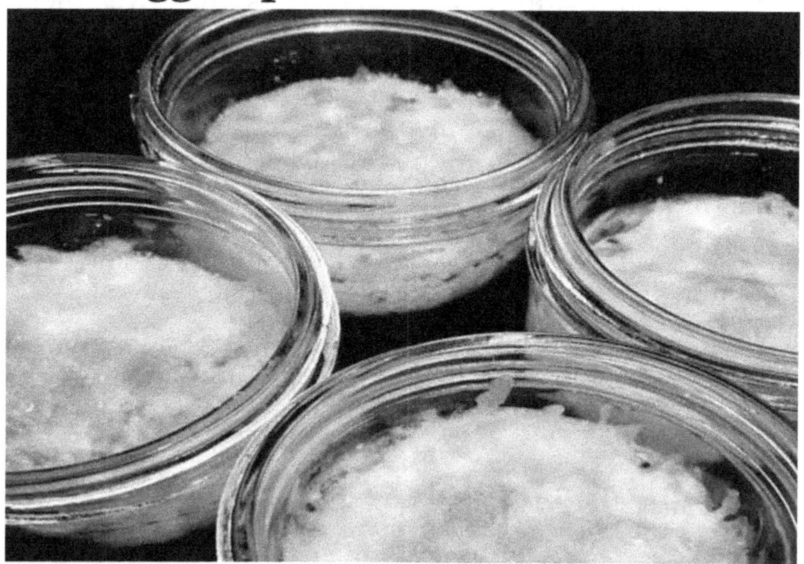

Prep time: 5 minutes
Cook time: 10 minutes
Servings: 4

Ingredients

- ½ cup of shredded cheddar cheese
- 4 large eggs
- Pepper and salt moderately to taste
- 2 tbsp finely chopped cilantro
- 1 cup diced veggies
- ¼ cup of half and half

Instructions

1. Mix all the ingredients together.
2. Divide the mixture into 4 containers and cover them. But don't tighten the containers so as to allow the eggs lose liquid.
3. Put about 2 cups of water in the pot and then a trivet above it.
4. Carefully position the egg jars on the trivet.
5. Set your instant pot on 'high pressure' and cook for 5 minutes. Then you can release the pressure.
6. Pour the half cup of cheese on it.
7. Place your eggs in an air fryer for 3 minutes to make the cheese melt.

Nutritional information

Calories: 115
Net carbs: 2g
Fat: 9g
Protein: 5g

Casserole

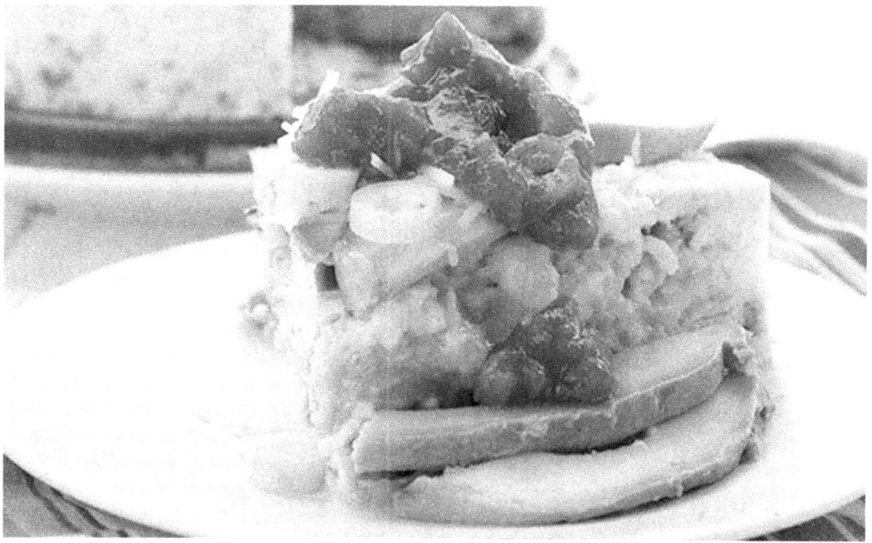

Prep time: 10 minutes

Cook time: 42 minutes

Servings: 6

Ingredients

- 2 tbsp avocado oil
- 1 well sliced green onion
- 1 cup of shredded cheese (Monterey Jack)
- 1 well sliced California Avocado
- Pepper and salt to taste
- 6 eggs
- 2 well-minced garlic cloves
- 3 grated broccoli stalks (medium preferable)
- 6 oz breakfast sausage
- Sour cream, more cheese and salsa for serving

Instructions

1. Get a casserole dish of about 7-inch diameter and grease it.
2. Set your instant pot on 'sauté'.
3. Add in the avocado oil.
4. Once the oil gets hot, add in the sausage and break into pieces with a hard spoon (preferably wooden spoon).
5. Cook for 4 minutes until there are no traces of pink in the pot remaining.
6. Properly mix the garlic, salt, pepper and broccoli stalks and then pour the mixture into the pot to cook for 2 minutes.
7. Pour the mixture into a baking dish.
8. Get a medium-sized bowl to combine the eggs and cream and thoroughly stir to combine well. Add in the green onions and cheese and then, stir again until the mixture is smooth.
9. Transfer the mixture in the pan and tightly cover the casserole dish.
10. Add a cup of water into the instant pot and then place a trivet on it.
11. Now, cautiously place the casserole dish on the set trivet and cover the pot.
12. After ensuring that the vent is also closed, set your instant pot to 'manual pressure' and the time to 35 minutes.
13. After cooking, allow natural release of pressure for 10 minutes.

14. After venting, take off the casserole dish from the instant pot.

15. Moderately top your breakfast with well sliced avocado and any other topping of your choice.

16. It is time for breakfast!

Nutritional information

Calories: 351

Net carbs: 6.8g

Protein: 18g

Fat: 28g

Broccoli Ham and Pepper Frittata

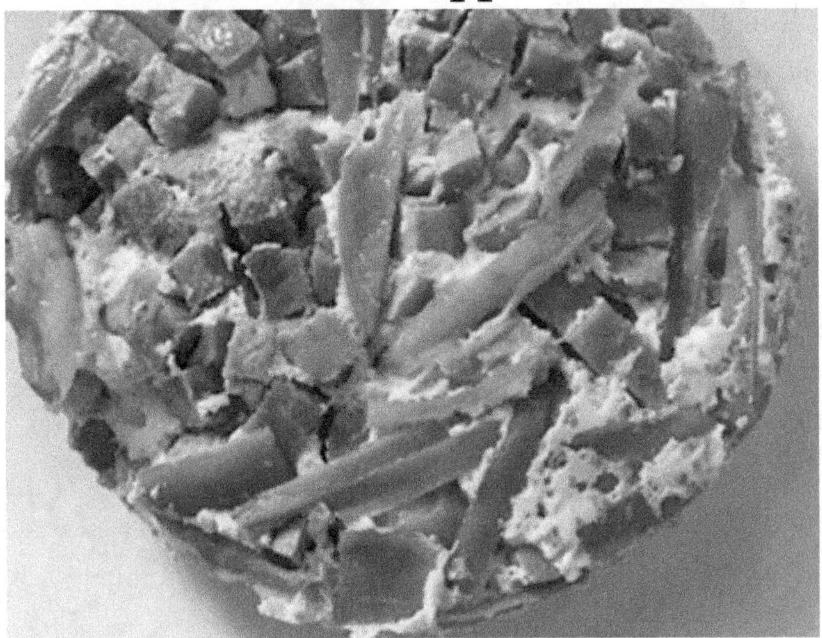

Prep time: 10 minutes
Cook time: 30 minutes
Servings: 4

Ingredients

- 8 oz cubed ham
- 4 large eggs
- 1 cup of sliced sweet peppers
- 2 cups of broccoli, frozen
- 1 cup of half and half
- Moderate amount of salt
- 2 tsp ground pepper
- 1 cup of cheddar cheese, shredded

Instructions

1. Take your time to thoroughly grease a 6-inch diameter pan. And I reiterate, thoroughly!
2. Place the sweet peppers on the lower part of the pan.
3. Then, the ham should be placed on the pepper.
4. Spread the broccoli over it. (NOTE: Fresh broccoli can perfectly work too).
5. Get a medium-sized bowl to mix the eggs, pepper, half and half and salt together. Stir very well to make them well-combined.
6. Add in the shredded cheese and mix well.
7. Pour egg mixture over the veggies and cover with a silicone lid.
8. Now, switch over to your instant pot: pour 2 cups of water in the liner.
9. Put a steamer rack on top of the water.
10. Now, you may carefully place the pan you covered with the silicone lid on the rack.
11. Set your pot on high pressure and cook for 20 minutes.
12. Let the pressure release naturally for 10 minutes before releasing the remaining on your own.
13. After about 10 minutes of sitting, use a knife to carefully loosen all the sides of your delicious meal. With a plate on the pan, the frittata can easily thump out on it.
14. If you don't want to serve it as it is, broil it for about 4 minutes and enjoy your healthy breakfast.

Nutritional information

Calories: 422
Net carbs: 7g
Fat: 30g
Protein: 24g

Poblano Cheese Frittata

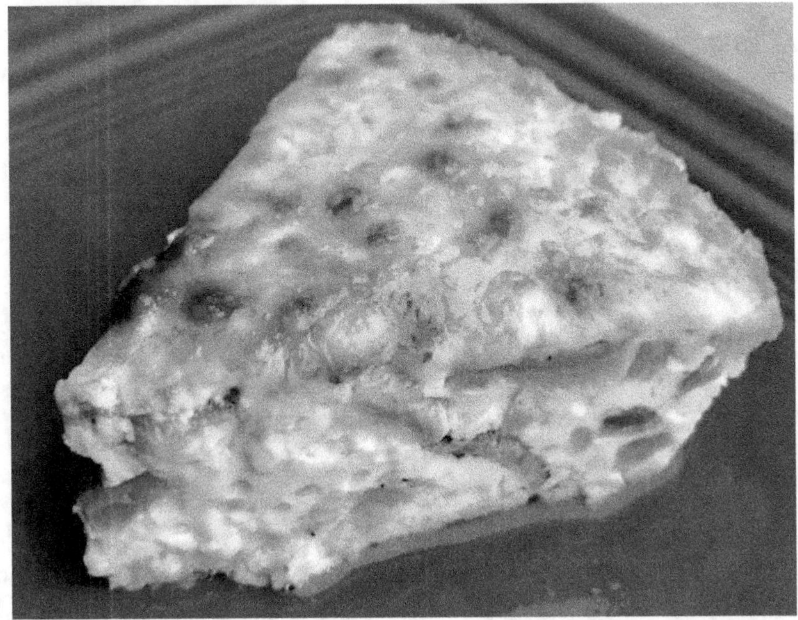

Prep time: 10 minutes
Cook time: 30 minutes
Servings: 4

Ingredients

- ¼ cup cilantro, finely chopped
- 4 large eggs
- 1 cup of half and half
- 10 oz green chiles, diced
- Salt to taste
- 1 cup of divided Mexican shredded cheese
- ½ tsp of ground cumin

Instructions

1. Crack eggs into a medium-sized bowl and add in half and half, chilis, salt, half portion of the shredded cheese and cumin. Mix until everything becomes smooth.
2. Thoroughly grease a 6-inch pan and pour the mixture into it, then cover it with foil.
3. Pour 2 cups of water into the inner liner of your instant pot and then place a trivet above the liner.
4. Gently put the pan over the trivet.
5. Set your pot on high pressure and cook for 20 minutes before releasing the pressure naturally (for 10 minutes).
6. Spread the remaining half portion of cheese on the quiche and broil for 5 minutes until it changes to brown.

Nutritional information

Calories: 257
Net carbs: 6g
Fat: 20g
Protein: 12g

Bacon and eggs muffins

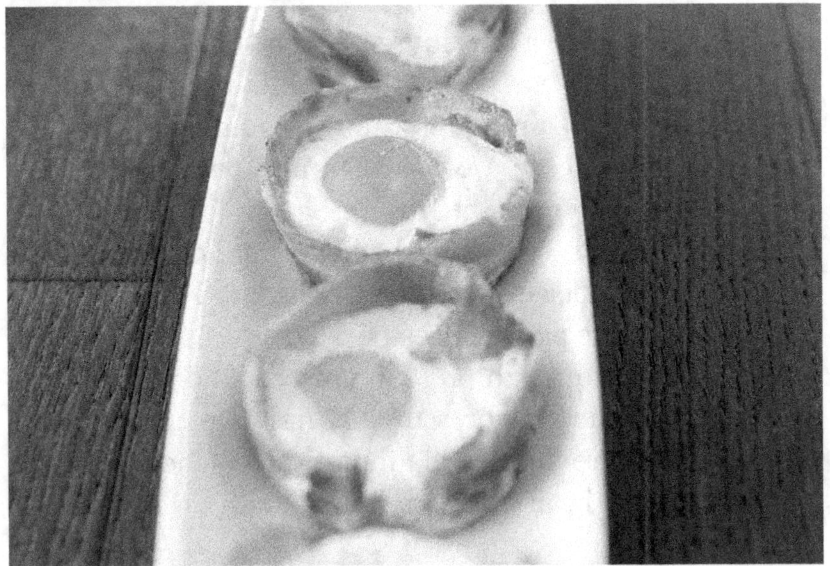

Prep time: 5 minutes

Cook time: 20 minutes

Servings: 2

Ingredients

- 4 eggs
- 8½ oz of bacon

Instructions

1. Cut the bacon into strips. Let it be long so as to serve as perfect casing for the muffins in the tray.
2. Cook until it turns brown. However, be careful of making them too crispy.
3. Properly dice the bacon you're left with in order to use them as a base. Don't worry if you're short of bacon; the eggs will perfectly play the role of a base.

4. Segment the muffin with the bacon.

5. Break an egg into each of the segments.

6. Cook for 10 minutes and your breakfast is ready!

Nutritional information

Calories: 700
Net carbs: 1g
Protein: 50g
Fat: 54g

Ground beef omelet

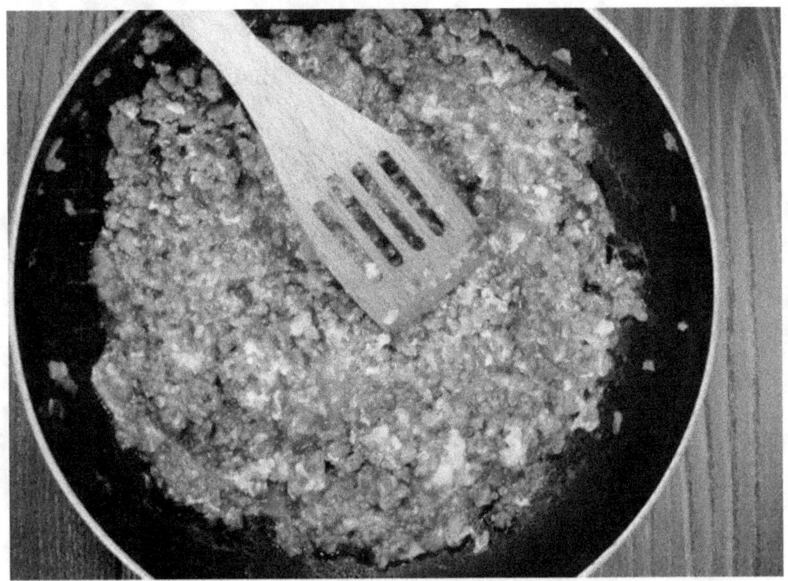

Prep time: 10 minutes
Cook time: 10 minutes
Servings: 2

Ingredients

- 1/4 cup of well chopped onions
- Salt to taste
- 3 beaten eggs
- 1 tbsp of oil
- ¼ tbsp ground black pepper
- 2 tbsp butter
- 7 oz of grass-fed lean ground beef

Instructions

1. Take out your big skillet and grease it properly. Heat with medium-high heat pressure.
2. Add in onion and let it fry for 2 minutes while you stir.

3. Add in the butter and let it completely melt.
4. Add in the beef and reset your pot to medium heat level.
5. With occasional stirring, cook for fifteen minutes.
6. Add salt, pepper and the eggs. Cook for a minute and stir well.
7. Remove your breakfast from heat and enjoy your delicious, healthy meal.

Nutritional information

Calories: 460
Net carbs: 1.7g
Fat: 32g
Protein: 37g

Avocado and egg fat bombs

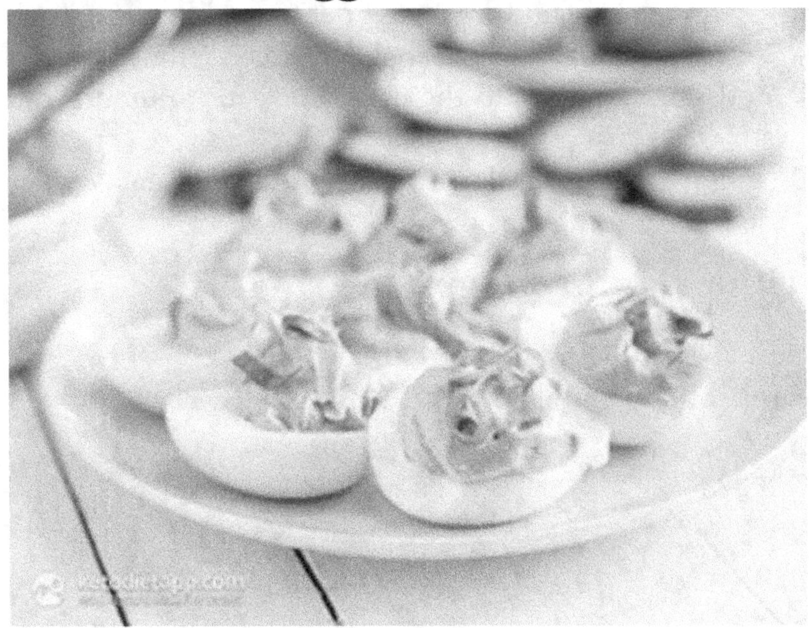

Prep time: 10 minutes
Cook time: 20 minutes
Servings: 3

Ingredients

- 3 boiled egg yolks
- 2 tbsp of finely chopped spring onions
- Black pepper, freshly ground
- 1 small avocado, with the seed removed and peeled
- 1 tbsp of lime juice
- Salt to taste, very moderate
- ¼ cup of mayonnaise

Instructions

1. Begin by boiling the eggs. Ensure there is plenty of water in the saucepan to prevent against egg cracking.

You may also add a pinch of salt to protect against cracking.

2. Use a spoon to take the eggs out of the boiling water. If you want a hard-boiled egg, set the timer to ten minutes.
3. Put in cold water in a medium-sized bowl and peel the shell off the eggs.
4. Divide the avocado into 2 equal halves and remove the seed. Then, peel the avocado.
5. Carefully halve the eggs, minding the yolks.
6. Use a spoon to empty the yolks into a medium-sized bowl.
7. Cut the avocado into tiny pieces. Add in the yolks, pepper, salt, mayonnaise and lemon juice.
8. Use a fork to smash the mixture until creamy and smooth.
9. Spread the spring onions to top it up. You can use the egg halves to make deviled eggs by filling them up.

Nutritional information

Calories: 147
Net carbs: 1.1g
Proteins: 2.2g
Fats: 14.8g

No Noodle Lasagna

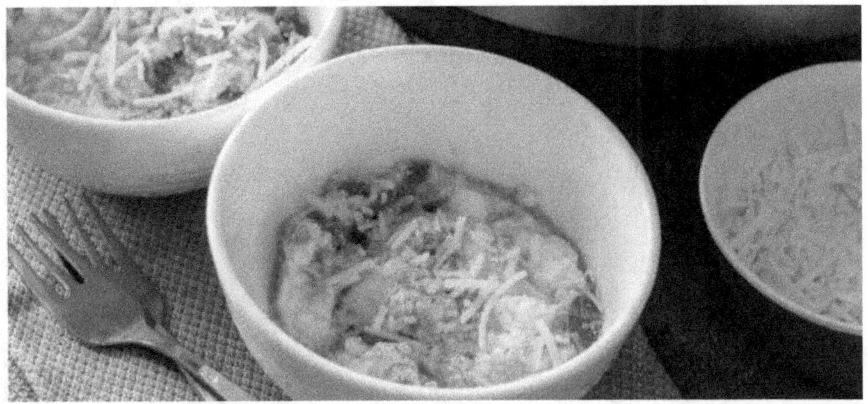

Prep time: 10 minutes
Cook time: 25 minutes
Servings: 8

Ingredients

- 1 onion
- 8 oz sliced mozzarella
- 1 egg
- 1 lb ground beef
- 2 minced garlic clove
- 25 oz jar of sauce
- 2 cups of ricotta cheese
- ½ cup parmesan cheese

Instructions

1. Set your instant pot on sauté to brown the beef, onion and garlic.
2. While the ground beef browns, get a small bowl to mix the Parmesan, ricotta cheese and eggs together. Stir very well to ensure they are well combined.

3. Take off the browned beef into a dish that aptly fits into an instant pot. 1 ½ quart soufflé dish would work well.
4. Divide the sauce into two. Add half to the beef and keep the remaining.
5. Halve the mozzarella cheese and add it to the meat sauce that is left.
6. Add half of the ricotta cheese on the mozzarella layer.
7. While reserving some pieces for the last layer, include another layer of mozzarella cheese on it.
8. Now, gently spread the remaining ricotta cheese over the mozzarella.
9. Add a cup of water to your instant pot and put the dish on the rack above the water. Cover the pot and use pressure cooking to cook for 10 minutes.
10. After venting off the steam, remove the lid and add the cheese. Sprinkling the parmesan cheese on the topmost part is one of my favorite ways of making this meal.
11. Now, it's time for serving!

Nutritional information

Calories: 365
Net carbs: 7g
Protein: 20g
Fat: 35g

Bacon Broccoli Frittata

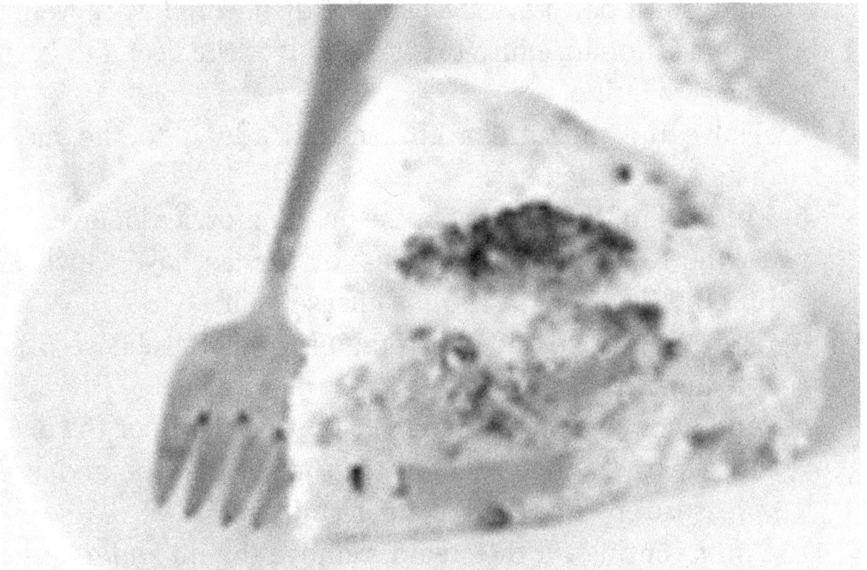

Prep time: 7 minutes
Cook time: 33 minutes
Servings: 6

Ingredients

- 2 tbsp grass-fed ghee
- A small piece of diced onion
- 4 eggs, pastured
- 4 finely minced clove garlic
- 1 cup of broccoli florets, finely chopped
- 1 tbsp of sea salt
- ¼ cup coconut milk
- 1 lemon
- 1 tbsp of fresh thyme, finely chopped
- 2 cups of cheddar cheese, shredded
- 1 cup of water

Instructions

1. Add in a fat of your choice and set your instant pot on sauté.
2. Once melted, add in the garlic and onion, and allow to sauté for 7 minutes. Then, you can add broccoli and allow to sauté for another 4 minutes.
3. Grease a casserole dish that can perfectly fit into your instant pot.
4. Get a medium-sized bowl to mix the eggs and milk together. Whisk until they're well-combined. Add in the sea salt, lemon, thyme and parsley (optional) and stir continuously until they are well incorporated.
5. Add in the cheese and garlic-onion mixture, and stir well to incorporate.
6. Transfer the well-combined mixture into the greased dish.
7. Pour the cup of water into the inner liner of the pot and place the trivet on it.
8. Gently place the dish on the trivet.
9. Ensure that the vent is sealed and cover the instant pot. Then, hit the 'manual' button of your pot and set the time to 23 minutes.
10. When it is done, let it release naturally for 10 minutes and quick release the remaining pressure. Then, you can uncover the pot.
11. Gently take out the casserole dish from the instant pot and you can either serve warm or hot!

Nutritional information

Calories: 162
Net carbs: 2.6g
Protein: 7.6g
Fat: 13.7g

Coconut Porridge

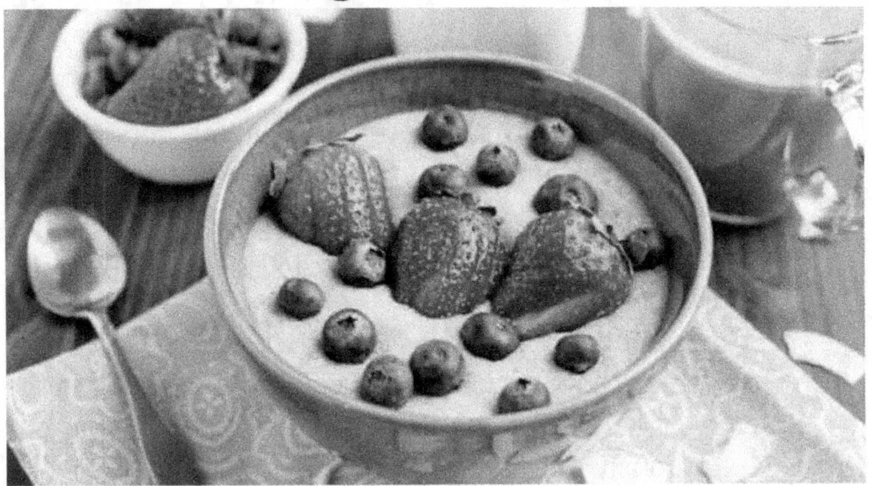

Prep time: 5 minutes

Cook time: 10 minutes

Servings: 6

Ingredients

- 1 cup of dried coconut, unsweetened
- 2 cups of coconut milk
- 20 drops each stevia and monk fruit liquids
- ¼ cup each coconut flour and psyllium husks
- ¼ tbsp nutmeg
- ½ tbsp. cinnamon
- 1 tsp of vanilla extract
- 3 cups of water

Instructions

1. Set your instant pot on sauté and toast the coconut until it turns golden. Don't let it burn.
2. Add in water and coconut milk. Then, stir continuously.
3. Set the timer of your pot to zero and cover the lid.
4. When it beeps, quickly release the pressure and uncover it.
5. Add in all other ingredients and stir to incorporate well.

Nutritional information

Calories: 303

Net carbs:5g

Protein: 6g

Fat: 29g

Philly Cheese Steak Wraps

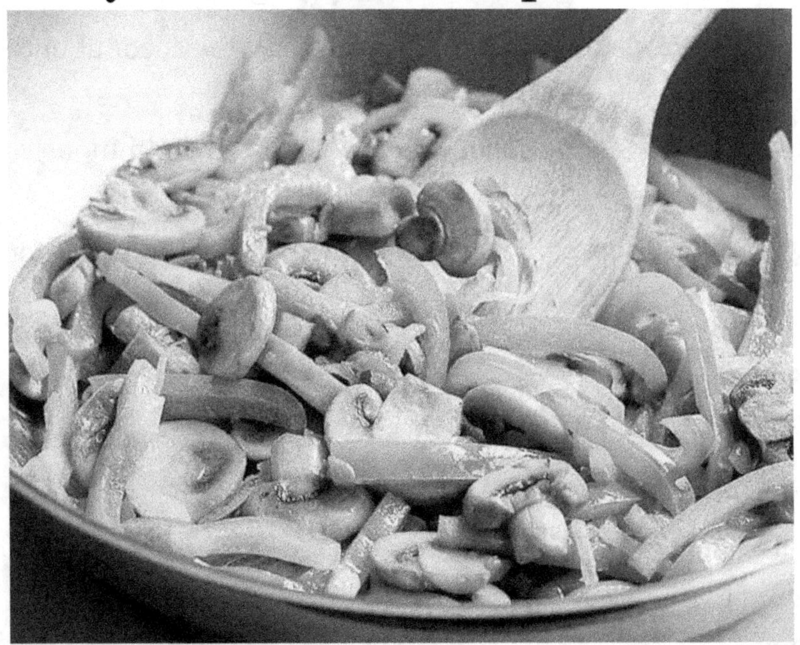

Prep time: 5 minutes
Cook time: 10 minutes
Servings: 4

Ingredients

- 8 oz of well sliced deli roast beef
- 4 oz of sliced Provolone cheese
- 2 tbsp olive oil
- 4 pieces of 1 oz green bell pepper
- 4 tortillas (almost zero carb wraps)
- 1 tbsp of Worcestershire sauce
- An inch of small sliced onion

Instructions

1. Turn your instant pot to medium pressure. Slice the green bell pepper and add to the pot, followed by the onions.
2. Reset your pot to sauté and add in the butter to melt for 2 minutes.
3. Add in the mushroom and stir well to incorporate. With occasional stirring, cook for 2 minutes.
4. Switch off the pot. Then, add in the Worcestershire sauce and roast beef. Set your pot to manual setting, and add in pepper and salt. Stir to combine well and cook for 3 minutes.
5. Take out the Philly steak mixture from the pot and add to two wraps.
6. To each wrap, add one-quarter of the steak mixture and a slice of cheese.
7. Seal the vent and use the lid to cover the pot. Let it cook for a minute and simmer. You may decide to release naturally or quick release the pressure.
8. Serve your delicious healthy breakfast!

Nutritional information

Calories: 445
Net carb: 3g
Proteins: 28g
Fats: 32g

Baking Eggs

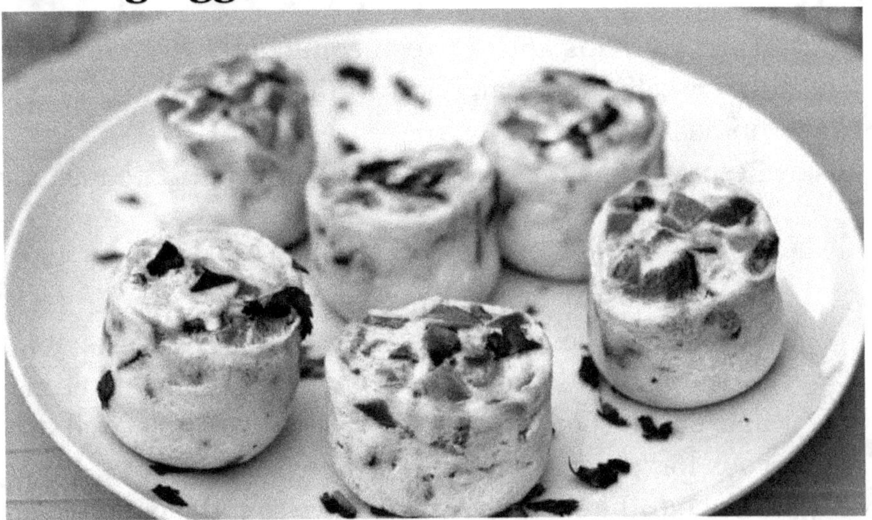

Prep time: 5 minutes
Cook time: 10 minutes
Servings: 4

Ingredients

- 6 large eggs
- 3 cooked bacon slices
- 1 tsp each of salt, cayenne and pepper
- ¼ cup crumbled feta cheese
- 2 minced clove garlic
- 1 cup of spinach, fresh
- 1 minced onion
- ½ cup heavy cream
- 1 cup of Italian cheese mozzarella, provolone, parmesan and Romano mix
- 8 oz of ground breakfast sausage

Instructions

1. Turn the instant pot to sauté. Brown the sausage.
2. During this process, add in seasoning, eggs, heavy cream and Italian cheese into a sizable bowl and mix until they all incorporate well.
3. Add in minced garlic and onion when the sausage is about to brown. Sauté for 3 minutes.
4. Switch off the sear key and put the spinach into the pot. Stir until it becomes somewhat wilted.
5. Add in spinach, sausage, onion and garlic mix to the egg mixture. Whisk and transfer the mixture into a properly greased bowl. Gently put crumbles of feta cheese onto the egg mix.
6. Clean your instant pot and pour a cup of water into it. Place a trivet on it and then, gently place the egg mixture on the set trivet.
7. Cover the pot and cook on high pressure for twenty minutes.
8. When it beeps, switch off the pressure cooker and let it release pressure naturally for 10 minutes.
9. Take out your breakfast egg bake and clean the top with a paper towel, in case steam has created moisture gather on it.
10. Top this delicious meal with the bacon or any topping you desire.

Nutritional information

Calories: 184
Net carbs: 2.5g
Fats: 14.4g
Proteins: 11.7g

Dairy Free Coconut Yogurt

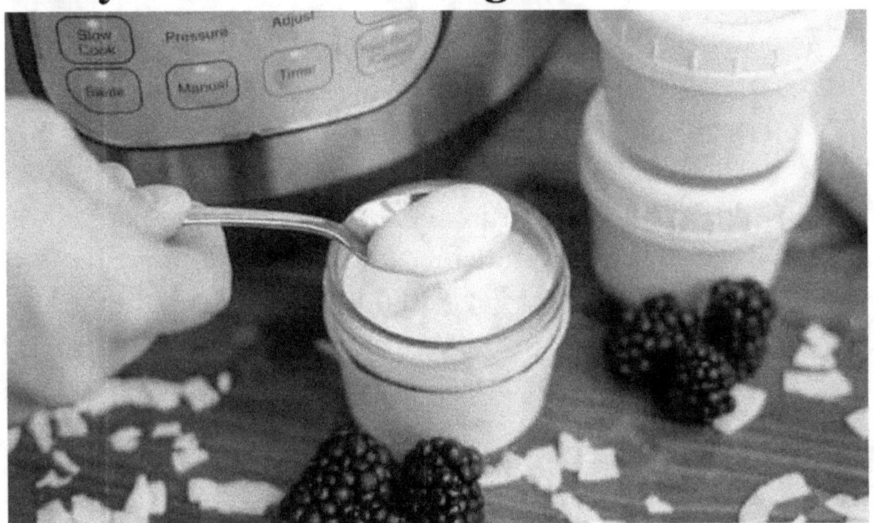

Prep time: 5 minutes

Cook time: 18 hours

Servings: 6

Ingredients

- 27 oz (2 cans) coconut cream
- Probiotic, 4 caps

Instructions

1. Add coconut cream into the pot.
2. Cover the pot and hit the 'yogurt' button on the instant pot.
3. Adjust the pot until it displays 'boil'.
4. When it beeps, uncover the instant pot and confirm if it has reached 115°F temperature.
5. Then, pour in the probiotic and whisk the mixture thoroughly.

6. Cover the pot again and reset it to 'Yogurt'. Set the timer to 16 to 18 hours.

7. When it beeps, uncover the pot. Transfer it into a container, cover and refrigerate for one day. By that time, it would have thickened up and would be ready for consumption.

Nutritional information

Calories: 420
Net carbs: 8g
Fats: 44g
Proteins: 4g

Pumpkin Pie Pudding

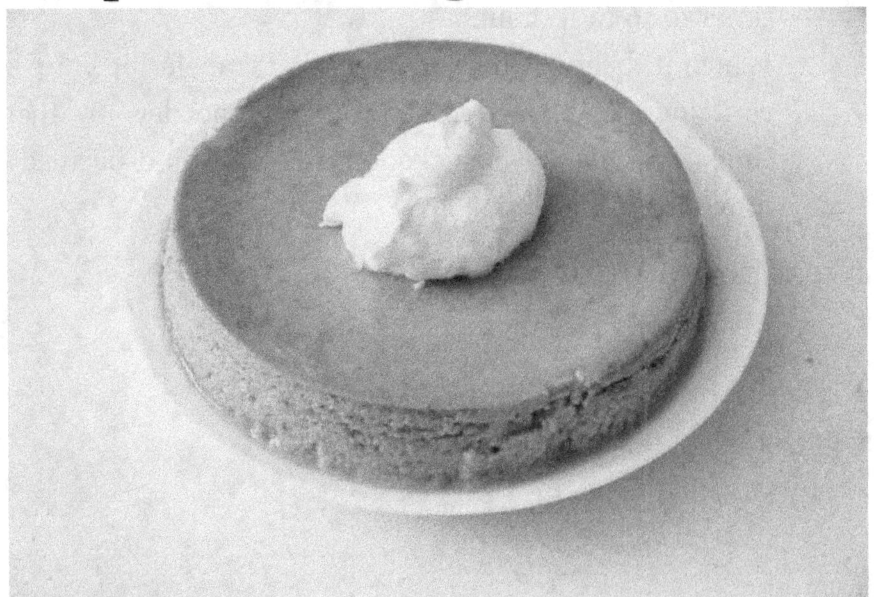

Prep time: 10 minutes
Cook time: 30 minutes
Servings: 6

Ingredients

- 2 large eggs
- ½ cup almond milk
- 1 tsp of pumpkin pie spice
- 15 oz pumpkin puree, canned
- 1 tsp vanilla extract
- ¾ cup of Erythritol

Instructions

1. Break the 2 eggs into a bowl and add all other ingredients.

2. Properly grease all sides of a pan (6-inches) and transfer the mixture into it.
3. Pour 1 ½ cups of water into the liner of the instant pot.
4. Put a steamer rack over the water and gently drop the pan on the rack.
5. Use aluminum foil or a silicone lid to cover the mixture pan.
6. Set your instant pot on high pressure and cook for 20 minutes. When it beeps, release the pressure naturally for 10 minutes before you do the quick release.
7. Carefully remove the lid without letting the water on it drop on the pudding.
8. Let it get cold for 7 hours and you can top up with extra heavy cream.

Nutritional information

Calories: 184
Net carbs: 8g
Proteins: 3g
Fats: 16g

Cauliflower and cheese

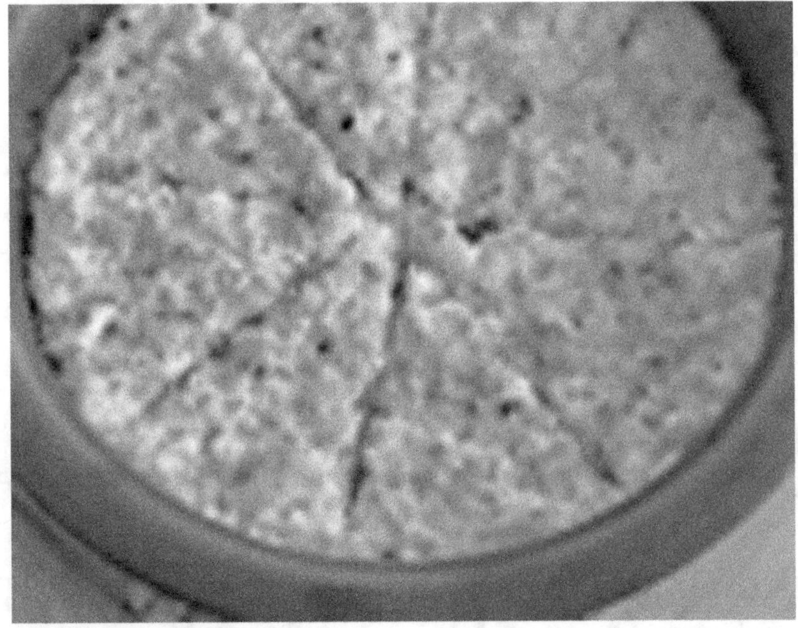

Prep time: 5 minutes
Cook time: 15 minutes
Servings: 2

Ingredients

- 2 cups of riced cauliflower
- ½ tsp each salt and ground pepper
- ½ cup of half and half
- 2 tbsp cream cheese
- 1/2 cup of sharp cheddar cheese, shredded

Instructions

1. Begin by mixing all the ingredients in a heatproof bowl.
2. Use a silicone lid or foil to cover the mixture.

3. Pour 1 ½ cups of water in the liner of the instant pot. Place a trivet on it and then gently place the mixture in the bowl on the trivet.
4. Let it cook on high pressure for 5 minutes and when it beeps, let it naturally release pressure for 10 minutes before you quick release the remaining pressure.
5. Put the cauliflower under the heated broiler to brown and bubble the cheese. It is time for serving!

Nutritional information

Calories: 270
Fats: 21g
Net carbs: 7g
Protein: 11g

Ketogenic Lunch

Spareribs

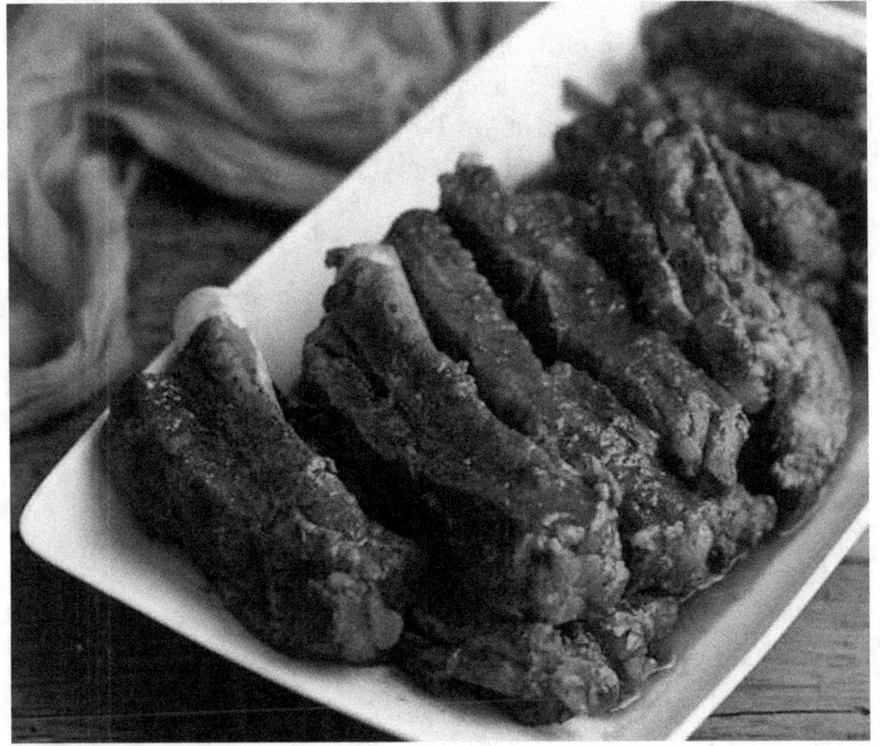

Prep time: 10 minutes
Cook time: 45 minutes
Servings: 6

Ingredients

- 5 lbs pork ribs, well cut into pieces

Dry rub

- 1 tsp each onion powder and paprika
- 1 ½ tbsp kosher salt
- 1 tsp garlic powder

- 1 tbsp of erythritol
- ½ tbsp of black pepper, *ground*
- ½ tsp of allspice
- ½ tsp of coriander, *ground*

Sauce

- ½ cup of water
- ½ tbsp ground allspice and mustard
- ½ tsp of onion powder
- ¼ tsp of liquid smoke
- 2 tbsp each of Red wine vinegar and erythritol
- ½ cup of reduced sugar ketchup

Instructions

1. Mix the dry rub ingredients together and use to whisk the ribs on every side.
2. Put the rib into your instant pot.
3. Mix all the sauce ingredients in a bowl and stir well. Then, pour the mixture over the ribs in the instant pot.
4. Seal the valve and cover the pot. Then, hit the high pressure button and set the cooking time to 35 minutes.
5. When it beeps, follow the manufacturer's guidelines to release pressure and uncover the pot.
6. Take out the ribs so as to platter.
7. Sauté the remaining liquid for 10 minutes and pour the ribs. It's serving time.

Nutritional information

Calories: 700
Net carbs: 3g
Protein: 100g
Fat: 70g

Shredded chicken

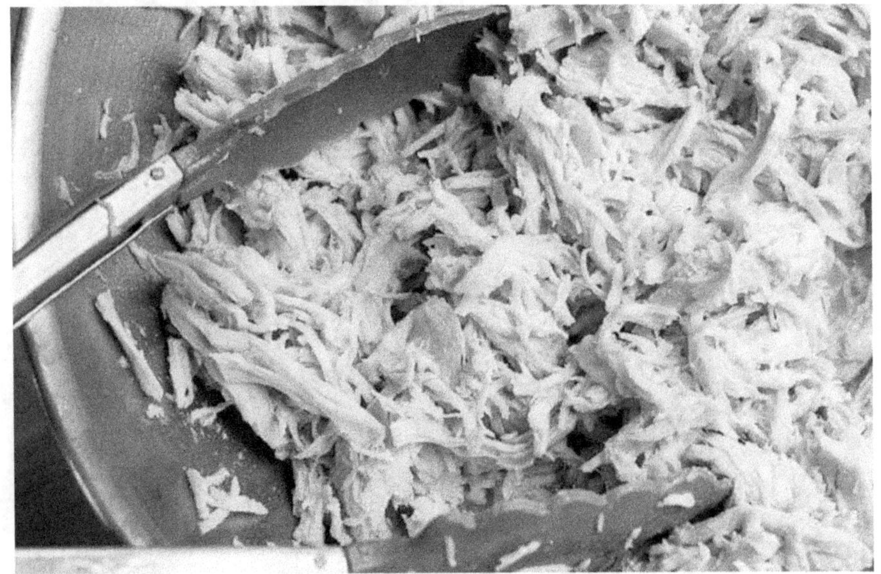

Prep time: 3 minutes

Cook time: 7 minutes

Servings: 12

Ingredients

- ¼ cup of chicken broth
- ¼ cup of refined coconut oil
- 3¾ lbs of chicken breast

Instructions

1. Put the chicken in the inner liner of the instant pot.
2. Add in the chicken broth and refined coconut oil.
3. Set the instant pot on high pressure and cook for 7 minutes.

4. When it is done cooking, take off the chicken from the pot and shred in a bowl.

5. Add desired amount of toppings and enjoy the yummy meal.

Nutritional information

Calories: 200

Net carbs: 1g

Fat: 10g

Protein: 30g

Bruschetta chicken with zoodles

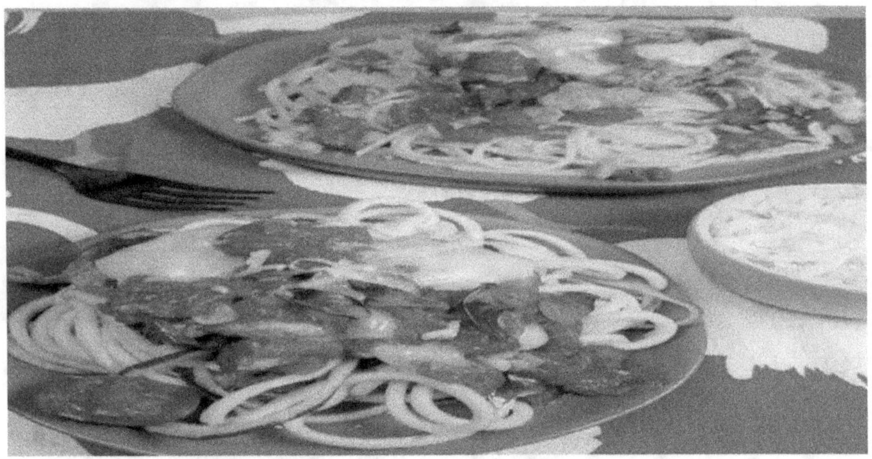

Prep time: 15 minutes
Cook time: 4 minutes
Servings: 4

Ingredients

- 4 boneless and skinless chicken breasts
- ½ cup of diced red onions
- ¼ cup of olive oil, extra virgin
- 2 ½ lbs of drained, diced tomatoes
- ¾ cup of grated fresh parmesan cheese
- 1 zucchini
- 8 oz of thinly sliced mozzarella cheese
- Minced and peeled fresh garlic
- ½ tsp of sea salt
- ½ tbsp basil leaves, fresh
- ¼ tsp of black pepper, ground
- 2 tbsp of balsamic vinegar
- 1 tbsp of chicken base

Instructions

1. Add in onion, chicken base, oil, garlic, vinegar, salt, pepper, chicken base and tomatoes to the instant pot and mix thoroughly.
2. Add in parmesan cheese and chicken.
3. Seal the valve and lock the lid of the instant pot. Hit the low pressure button and cook for 3 minutes. When it beeps, let it naturally release for 5 minutes.
4. Prepare zoodles.
5. Uncover the pot and add in the basil.
6. Put the chicken on zoodles. Spread the mozzarella cheese on the chicken and sprinkle the bruschetta over it.

Nutritional information

Calories: 118
Net carbs: 1.3g
Protein: 3g
Fat: 12.7g

Crack chicken

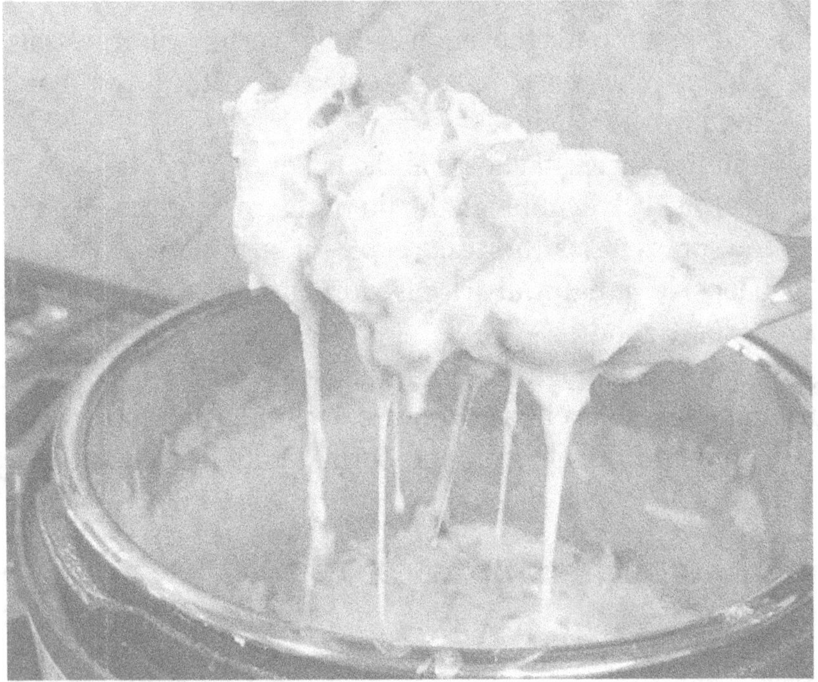

Prep time: 10 minutes
Cook time: 17 minutes
Servings: 8

Ingredients

- 2 lbs boneless and skinless chicken breasts
- 12 oz of cream cheese
- 8 oz of bacon crumbles
- ½ cup of cheddar cheese
- 1 cup of bone broth (water can work too)
- 1 oz packet Dry ranch seasoning mix, 2 pieces (homemade version is the best for you as a *keto-er*)

Instructions

1. Pour a cup of bone broth or water into the instant pot.
2. Divide the blocks of cream cheese into cubes (make them a bit large).
3. Put the chicken into the instant pot.
4. Then, add in the seasonings and cream cheese. Set your pot to high pressure cooking and allow it to cook for 12 minutes.
5. Once it beeps, quick release the pressure.
6. Take out the chicken with caution and use 2 forks to shred it in a large bowl and return in to the instant pot.
7. Now, add in the bacon crumbles and cheddar cheese and stir well. Cover the pot again and let it sit for 5 minutes.
8. It's time to enjoy your healthy meal.

Nutritional information

Calories: 392
Net carbs: 1.2g
Protein: 37g
Fat: 25.6g

Pork and Kraut

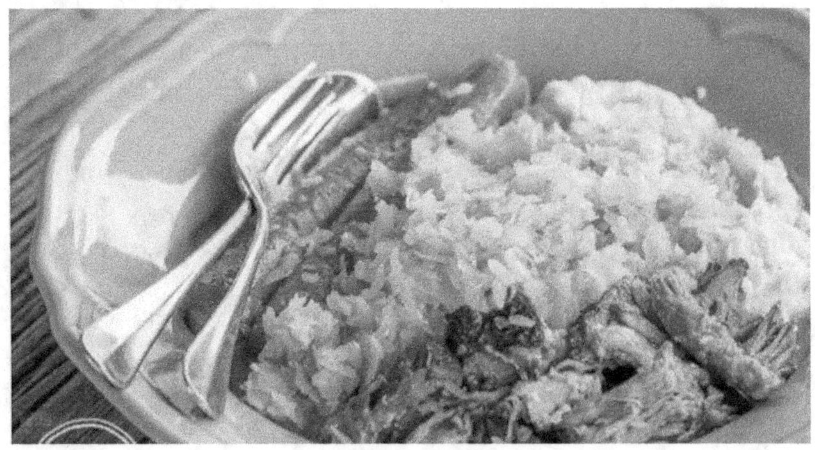

Prep time: 15 minutes
Cook time: 45 minutes
Servings: 6

Ingredients

- 3 lbs pork roast
- 2 finely chopped onions
- 2 tbsp of coconut oil, organic
- 6 cups of divided sauerkraut
- 1 lb of nitrate-free hot dogs (optional)
- ½ lb nitrate-free kielbasa (optional)
- Salt to taste
- 1 cup of filtered water
- 3 peeled and sliced garlic cloves
- 1/4 tsp of ground black pepper

Instructions

1. Whisk the pork with pepper and salt and put aside.
2. Heat a skillet on a high heat, and pour the coconut oil in it. Brown the pork on every side.

3. Transfer the pork roast to the rack of your instant pot and add in water, onion and garlic. Again, add some pepper and sea salt.
4. Cook on the high pressure for 35 minutes and let it naturally release pressure when it beeps.
5. Then add in half portion of the sauerkraut.
6. Reset the pot to high pressure and cook the kraut and pork for 5 minutes. Then quick release the pressure.
7. If you want the kielbasa and hot dogs, add them at this point and cook for another 5 minutes and quick release the pressure.
8. Top with the remaining raw kraut and enjoy this special meal.

Nutritional information

Calories: 350
Net carbs: 5g
Protein: 25g
Fat: 20g

Bacon Hash

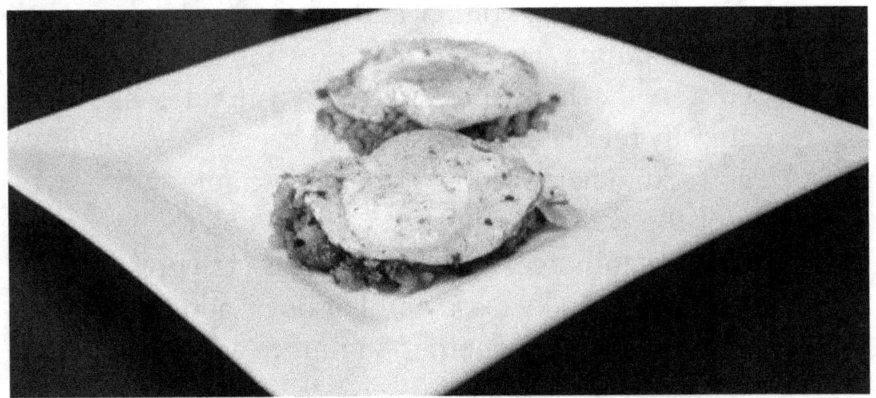

Prep time: 10 minutes
Cook time: 20 minutes
Servings: 2

Ingredients

- Slices of Jalapenos, well diced
- 4 large eggs
- Onion and pepper, very minimal
- Bacon, 6 slices
- 1 cup of water

Instructions

1. Set the instant pot to sauté and put the bacon in insert to cook to crisp. When it is done cooking, remove the grease and lay the bacon slices on the spring-form pan.
2. Let the jalapenos be well diced and then brown all sides.
3. Mix all the ingredients in a bowl and pour the mixture in the pan. Use foil to cover the pan.
4. Pour a cup of water in the liner of the pot and place a trivet on it. Gently place the pan on the trivet.

5. Seal the valve and lock the lid of the pot. Let it cook on pressure for 15-20 minutes. When it beeps, let it release pressure naturally.
6. Remove the foil from the pan and use a knife to slide the edges of the pan so as to remove eggs that would have been stuck there.
7. You may top the hash with some green onion and cheddar cheese.

Nutritional information

Calories: 366
Net carbs: 7g
Fat: 24g
Protein 23g

Cobb salad

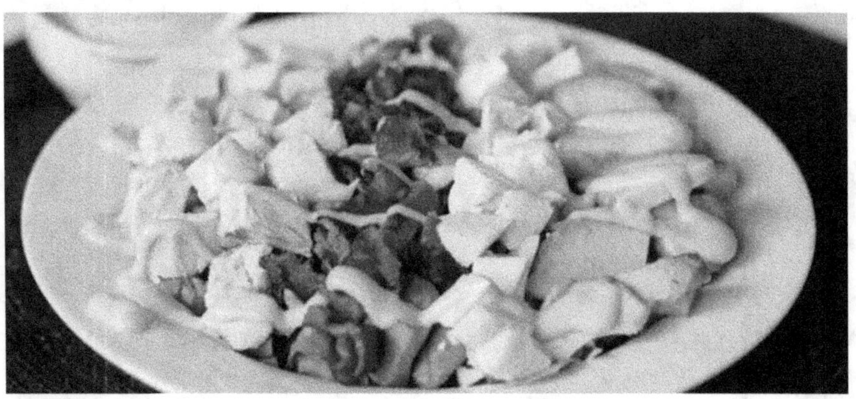

Prep time: 10 minutes
Cook time: 15 minutes
Servings: 4

Ingredients

For salad

- 1 Haas avocado
- 8 oz of cooked chicken
- 2 eggs, free range
- 4 cups of Romaine lettuce, well-chopped
- 4 uncured bacon

Dressing

- A piece of Haas avocado
- A pressed garlic clove
- 3 tbsp of extra virgin olive oil
- 1/3 cup of coconut milk
- 1 tbsp lemon juice
- ¼ tsp of sea salt
- 1 tbsp of organic Dijon mustard
- 1 tbsp of champagne vinegar, organic

Instructions

1. Pour water into saucepan to submerge eggs. Let it simmer for 15 minutes. After chilling, peel and dice the eggs.
2. Heat the medium pressure button to cook the bacon in a skillet. Carefully dice the cooked chicken.
3. Prepare the dressing by blending all the ingredients together and add some water.
4. Expertly chop the lettuce share among the bowls for serving.
5. Add in chicken, bacon, egg and diced avocado to the serving bowl. Sprinkle the dressing on it.

Nutritional information

Calories: 474
Net carbs: 4g
Proteins: 24g
Fat: 39g

Chicken foot broth

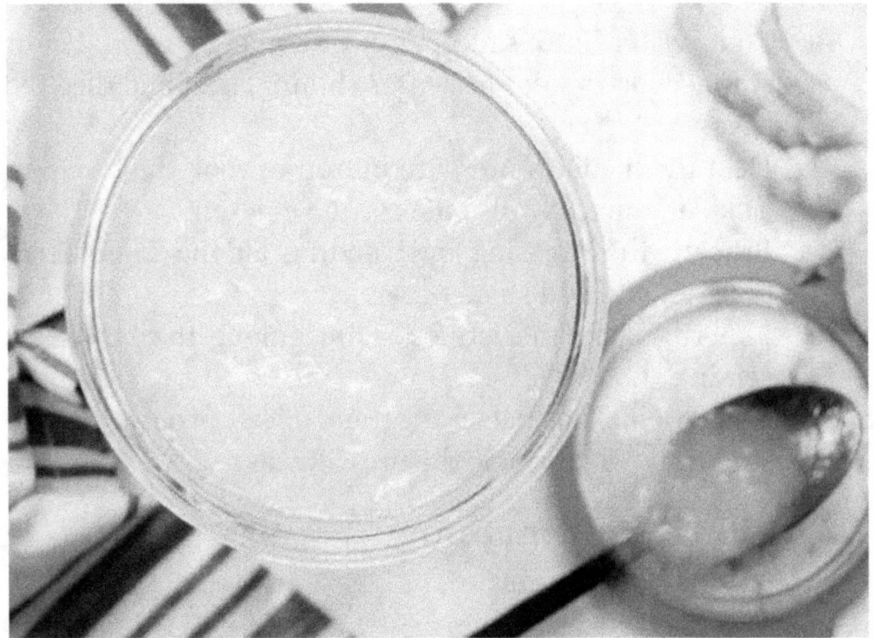

Prep time: 10 minutes

Cook time: 90 minutes

Servings: 4

Ingredients

- 15 peeled chicken feet
- 1 cup filtered water
- ¼ cup of apple cider vinegar

Instructions

1. Put the chicken feet in the insert of the instant pot.
2. Add in water to the pot so that it covers the chicken and then, add the cider vinegar.

3. Seal the valve and cover the pot with its lid. Hit the manual button and set the time to 90 minutes pressure cooking.

4. When it's done, allow it to naturally release pressure or you quick release the pressure.

5. Remove the broth from the feet and your meal is ready.

Nutritional information

Calories: 582

Net carbs: 5.6g

Protein: 35g

Fat: 14.5g

Mexican-style Pork Shoulder Tacos

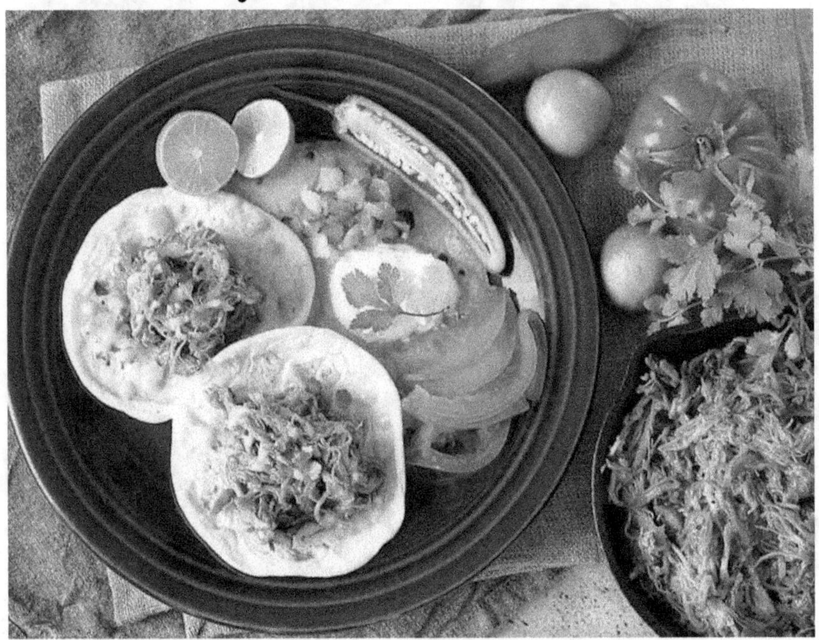

Prep time: 45 minutes
Cook time: 30 minutes
Servings: 6

Ingredients

- 1 tbsp of splenda
- 1 tsp each of onion and garlic powders
- 1 tsp each for smoked paprika and cumin, ground
- Salt, moderately to taste
- ¼ cup of water
- ½ tsp black pepper
- 1/2 tsp of ancho chile powder
- 1 ½ lbs boneless pork shoulder
- 4 lbs pork roast

Instructions

1. Mix all the ingredients properly in a large bowl.
2. Add in the pork into the instant pot and pour the spice rub on it. Then, let it marinate for half an hour.
3. Transfer the pork into the inner liner of the pot.
4. Pour in the ¼ cup of water.
5. Set your instant pot on high pressure manual and let it cook for 25 minutes. When it beeps, let it release pressure naturally for 10 minutes. After that, you may release any remaining pressure.
6. After shredding the pork shoulder, return to the cooking mixture until you're ready to serve.
7. You may serve with taco fixings if you so desire.

Nutritional information

Calories: 157
Net carbs: 1.4g
Proteins: 20g
Fat: 15g

Mustard, Tarragon and chicken soup

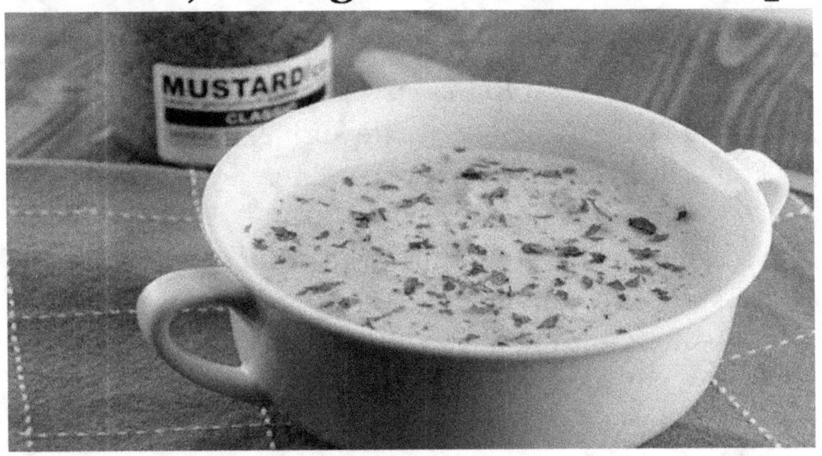

Prep time: 10 minutes
Cook time: 90 minutes
Servings: 4

Ingredients

- 4 boneless and skinless chicken thighs
- 4 tbsp of butter
- 4 oz of cream cheese
- 1 ½ tsp of tarragon
- ¼ tsp each onion and garlic powders,
- Pepper and salt moderately to taste
- 1 cup of coconut milk
- 1 cup of heavy whipping cream
- 1 tsp of mustard

Instructions

1. Sprinkle the chicken thighs with pepper and salt.
2. Use the medium-high heat setting to heat the coconut oil.

3. Cook the chicken thighs in the oil and turn periodically so as to make all the sides brown. This should be done for 3 minutes. Then, remove from oil and put in a plate.
4. Drain the pot of oil and add in the butter; heat by turning the instant pot to medium-high heat setting.
5. Add in the tarragon.
6. Add in the browned chicken and seal the vent, lock the lid and cook for 10 minutes at high pressure.
7. When it beeps, follow the manufacturer's manual to quick release pressure.
8. Now, you can put the chicken in a serving bowl, cover with an aluminum foil to ensure it's warm.
9. Mix every other left ingredient in a bowl and add in to the instant pot. Cook until it becomes thick to your desired taste.
10. Add in the chicken again to coat properly and it's ready to be served.

Nutritional information

Calories: 504
Net carbs: 1.7g
Proteins: 16.5g
Fat: 49.5g

Cauliflower Soufflé

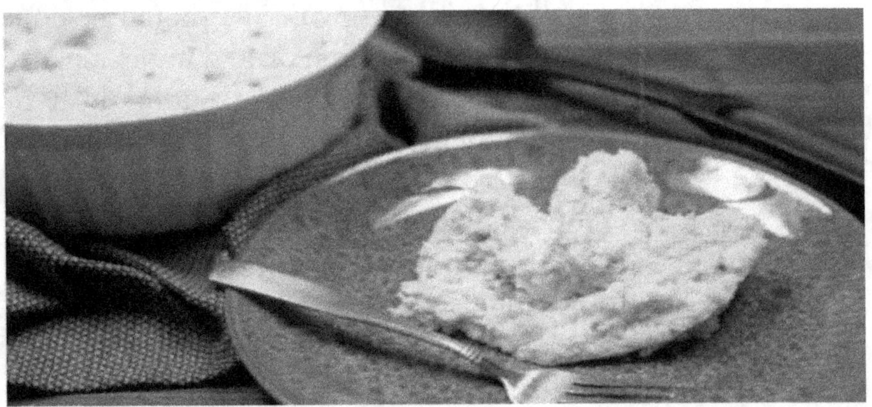

Prep time: 10 minutes
Cook time: 20 minutes
Servings: 6

Ingredients

- A head of cauliflower
- 2 large eggs
- 2 oz of cream cheese
- ½ cup each sour cream and Asagio cheese
- 2 tbsp soft butter
- ¼ cup of chives
- 1 cup of mild cheddar cheese
- 2 packets of TBL cream
- 6 slices of cooked and crumbled 'no sugar bacon' (Optional)

Instructions

1. Put eggs, cheddar cheese, cream, Asagio and sour cream in a food processor. Process until the mixture becomes frothy and smooth.

2. Chop cauliflower finely, add to mixture and stir thoroughly. Add in the butter and chives.
3. Grease all the sides and corners of a casserole dish and transfer the mixture into it.
4. Pour a cup of water in the inner liner of the instant pot and place the trivet above it. Then, carefully put the dish on the trivet.
5. Seal the valve and lock the lid of the pot. Let it cook on high pressure for 12 minutes and when it beeps, allow it to release pressure naturally for another 10 minutes.
6. Take out the dish and you can serve with cooked and crumbled bacon if you like.

Nutritional information

Calories: 342
Net carbs: 5g
Proteins: 17g
Fat: 28g

Arroz Con Pollo

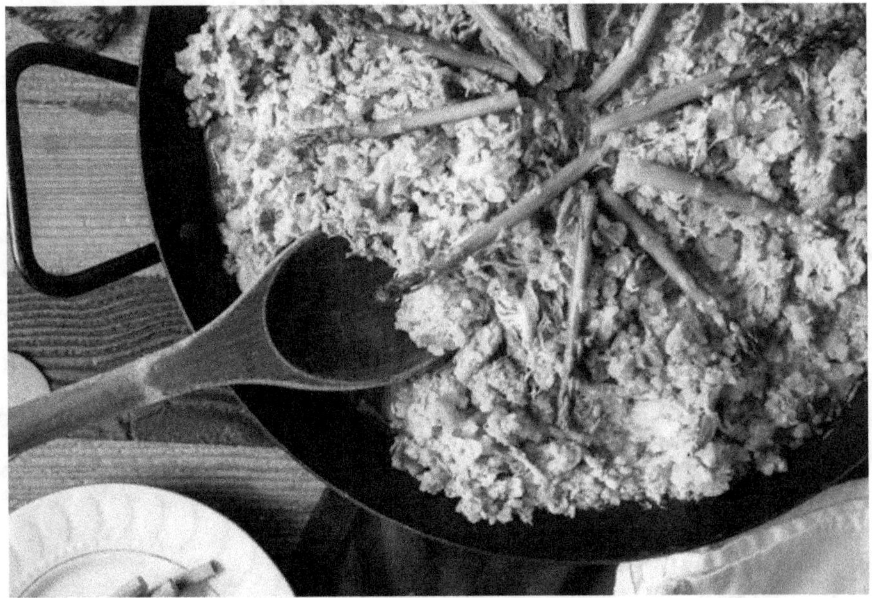

Prep time: 10 minutes
Cook time: 35 minutes
Servings: 8

Ingredients

- 3 slices of sugar-free and nightshade-free bacon
- 3 lbs chicken thighs, boneless and skinless
- 1 onion and 2 bay leaves
- 3 carrots, medium size
- 4 cloves garlic
- 1 cup diced of stalk rhubarb
- ¼ tsp olive oil and red wine vinegar
- 1 tbsp dried oregano
- 1 tsp sea salt
- 1 tbsp celery salt
- 1 tbsp garlic powder
- 24 oz frozen cauliflower rice (2 bags)

- 1 tsp turmeric
- 1 cup of bone broth
- Asparagus (optional)

Instructions

1. Set your instant pot on sauté to heat. While it is heating up, dice the onion, carrot, garlic, rhubarb and bacon.
2. Once it heats, add in the bacon and stir occasionally until it is cooked. Pour the other diced veggies and the bay leave in the pot. Stir thoroughly so that everything is well mixed. Let it cook for 8 minutes.
3. The chicken thighs may now go in. stir once in a while so that all sides of the chicken can become brown. Pour every seasoning into the pot and stir properly.
4. Add in the olive oil and vinegar. Seal the valve and close the pot. Let it cook on high pressure for 20 minutes after hitting the 'poultry' button.
5. When it beeps, let it release pressure naturally and then, unlock the lid. Add in the bone broth and cauliflower rice.
6. Cover the pot and allow it cook on low pressure for 3 minutes. After that, manually release the pressure.
7. After tasting, you may add some salt to taste. You may also decide to top it with steamed Asparagus.

Nutritional information

Calories: 337
Net carbs: 2.2g
Proteins: 45g
Fat: 16g

Chinese chicken and broccoli

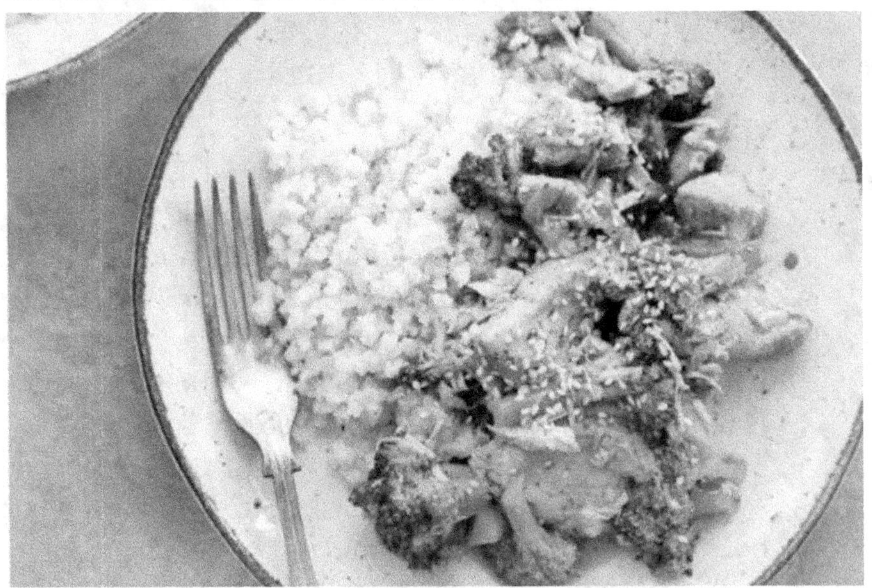

Prep time: 5 minutes
Cook time: 10 minutes
Servings: 2

Ingredients

- 1 lb boneless and skinless chicken thigh
- ¼ tsp Black pepper and sea salt
- ½ cup of chicken broth
- 1/4 cup of coconut aminos
- 1 tsp fish sauce
- 2 tbsp sesame oil
- 2 tbsp each Arrowroot and water
- ¼ tsp of apple cider vinegar
- 2 minced clove garlic
- 11-in crushed knob ginger
- 6 cups of broccoli florets
- 1 cup slurry

- Red pepper flakes (optional)
- Garnishing: sesame seeds

Instructions

1. Put chicken in the insert segment of the instant pot.
2. Add in sesame oil, coconut amino, pepper, garlic, ginger, salt and fish sauce.
3. Set the pot on manual and cook on high pressure for 8 minutes.
4. When it beeps, quick release the pressure.
5. Pour in slurry and combine well by stirring.
6. Press the cancel/warm button and switch to sauté. It's time to place the broccoli and let it sauté for another 5 minutes. Stir occasionally until the broccoli becomes soft and the liquid gets thickened.
7. Pour in the apple cider vinegar to bring out the flavor. Garnish with sesame seeds and serve with either white rice or cauliflower rice.

Nutritional information

Calories: 477
Net carbs: 13g
Fat: 30g
Protein: 45g

Tastes like pie chicken

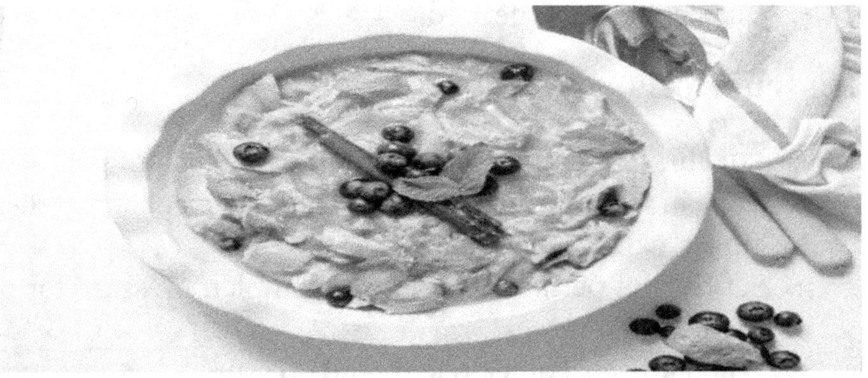

Prep time: 10 minutes
Cook time: 40 minutes
Servings: 4

Ingredients

- 2 lbs chicken thighs, boneless and skinless
- 1 Vidalia medium-sized onion
- 1 tbsp minced turmeric root
- 2 tsp each lemon juice and coconut aminos
- 1 clove garlic, smashed
- 2 tsp smoked salt
- 2 tbsp organic palm oil
- 1 cinnamon stick
- 3 mint sprigs
- ½ tbsp fresh blueberries
- 1 tbsp coconut flour

Instructions

1. Sauté the instant pot.

2. Pour the organic palm oil shortening into the pot and slice the onion. Also mince the turmeric root about an inch.

3. Add in the turmeric and onion to the instant pot. Stir from time to time and allow them to brown.

4. Pour the flour into the pot and mix thoroughly.

5. Season the chicken thighs with salt and then drop it into the instant pot. After stirring properly, add in the lemon, garlic, coconut aminos and stick cinnamon. Do not forget to give it a good stirring.

6. Reset the pot to pressure cooking and press the poultry button. Let it cook for 20 minutes.

7. When it beeps, let it release pressure and then, unlock the lid. Change the pot's setting to 'reduce'. Stir once in a while as it reduces for 10 minutes.

8. Add in blueberries and top your yummy meal with mint. What else? Serving!

Nutritional information

Calories: 498
Net carbs: 1.3g
Fat: 24g
Protein: 65g

Garlic Herb Pulled Chicken

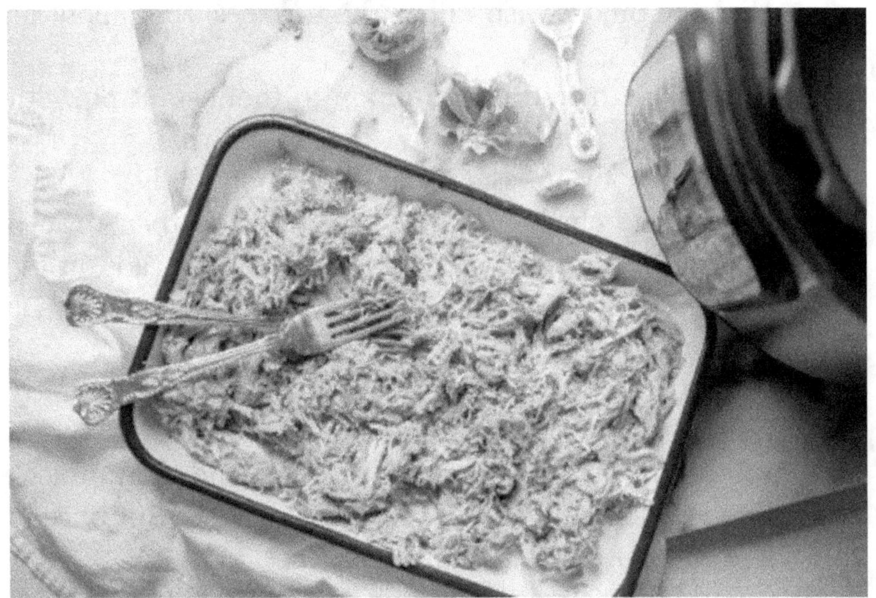

Prep time: 5 minutes
Cook time: 15 minutes
Servings: 7

Ingredients

- 2 lbs chicken thighs, boneless and skinless
- Black pepper (moderately to taste)
- 3 minced cloves garlic
- 1 peeled yellow onion
- ½ tbsp each dried basil and dried thyme
- ½ tsp sea salt
- 3/4 cup of water
- ½ tbsp of dried oregano

Instructions

1. Pour the water into your pot and add in the yellow onion, sliced and cut into rings.
2. Mix oregano, salt, pepper and thyme in a bowl and stir well.
3. Use the mixture to season the chicken in all sides. After that, lay the chicken on the onions in the pot.
4. Pour garlic on the seasoned chicken.
5. Seal the valve and cover the instant pot. Click on the poultry button and let it cook for 15 minutes.
6. When it beeps, turn the valve to vent so as to quick release pressure.
7. After releasing pressure, take out the chicken into a bowl.
8. Use 2 forks to shred the chicken.
9. You may add some of the broth to your chicken for moisture or enjoy it as it is.

Nutritional information

Calories: 267
Net carbs: 1.8g
Fat: 13g
Proteins: 33g

Ketogenic Dinner

Avocado Egg Salad

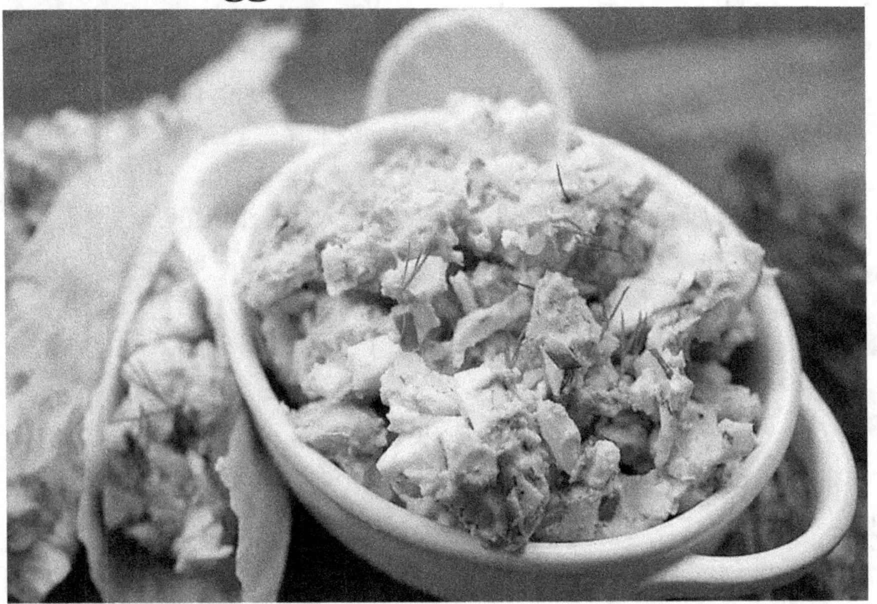

Prep time: 5 minutes
Cook time: 5 minutes
Servings: 6

Ingredients

- 6 large eggs, boiled
- 2 diced avocado
- ½ tsp each pepper and salt
- 2 tsp dill, fresh
- ¼ cup of red onion, well-minced
- 1 lemon

Instructions

1. Boil the eggs in your pot for 5 minutes with the high pressure cooker. Make sure that the water reaches ¾ of the pot to prevent cracking.
2. Allow the pot to release pressure naturally for another 5 minutes and quick release the remaining pressure. Then, transfer the eggs into an ice bath for another 5 minutes and you're done with the cooking stage.
3. Peel the eggs into a medium-sized bowl and dice them.
4. Add in the two diced avocado and stir thoroughly to make it coat the diced eggs when it breaks down.
5. Squeeze your lemon on the combined mixture and add every other ingredient. Take your time to stir until they become well combined.
6. Serve right away!

Nutritional information

Calories: 155
Net carbs: 3g
Fat: 12g
Protein: 5.7g

Smothered Pork Chops

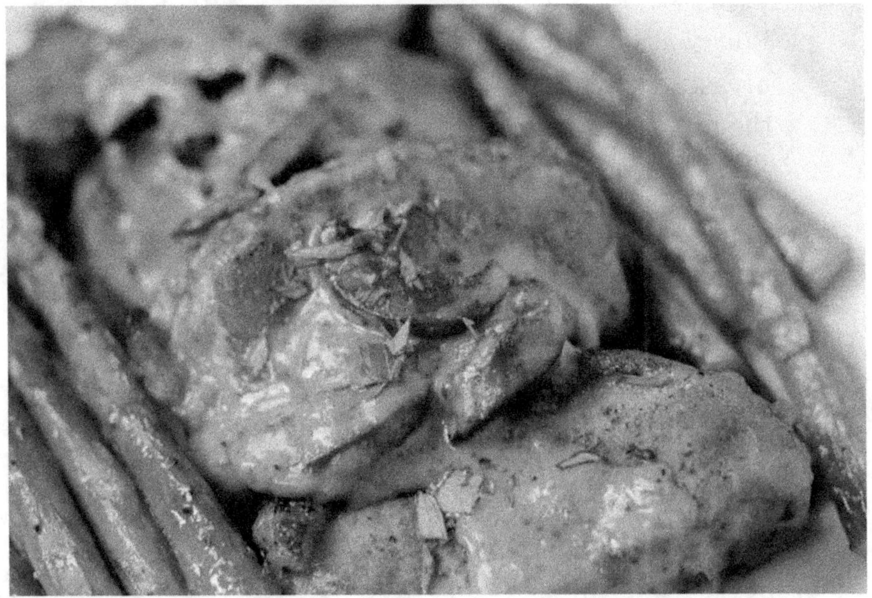

Prep time: 10 minutes
Cook time: 40 minutes
Servings: 4

Ingredients

- 6 oz loin chops boneless pork
- 1 tbsp paprika
- 1 tbsp each black pepper and salt
- 1 tsp garlic and onion powders
- 2 tbsp coconut oil
- 1 small sliced onion
- 1 tbsp freshly chopped parsley
- ½ tbsp xanthan gum
- ½ cup heavy whipping cream
- 6 oz baby bella mushroom, sliced
- 1 tbsp butter
- ¼ tbsp cayenne pepper

Instructions

1. Properly mix the garlic, salt, black pepper, onion powder and cayenne powder in a medium-sized bowl.
2. Use water to rinse the chops and pat. Spray the sides of the pork chops with a tablespoonful of the mixture (spice) and carefully rub the seasoning into the inner part of the meat. Put the remaining spice mixture aside.
3. Set your instant pot on saute and heat the coconut oil.
4. Put the pork chops in the heated oil to brown (after three minutes, turn the other side too to brown for 3 minutes). Then, you can take it off the oil and turn of your Instant pot.
5. Add in your well-sliced onions and mushrooms to the base of the pot. The pork chops can now follow.
6. Seal the vent of the pot, cover the pot and hit the Manual High button and cook for 25 minutes. When it beeps, you may decide to release the pressure manually or through natural means.
7. Put the pork chops on a serving plate and uncover the pot.
8. Reset your pot to sauté. Add in the heavy cream, butter and the spice mixture you're left with in the hot liquid.
9. Divide the xanthan gum into 2 ½ and add a half into the mixture and stir thoroughly. Let it simmer for 5 minutes so as to allow the butter melt and the sauce become thick.
10. Switch off the instant pot and add the remaining xanthan gum for the gravy to become thick to your desired taste. In some instances, you may need more. Also take cognizance of the fact that the gravy becomes thicker as it gets cold.
11. Add mushroom gravy and onion to the pork chops. Spread the parsley on it and it's time to serve!

Nutritional information

Calories: 481.25
Net carbs: 4.06g
Protein: 14.75g
Fat: 32.61g

Garlic 'butter' chicken

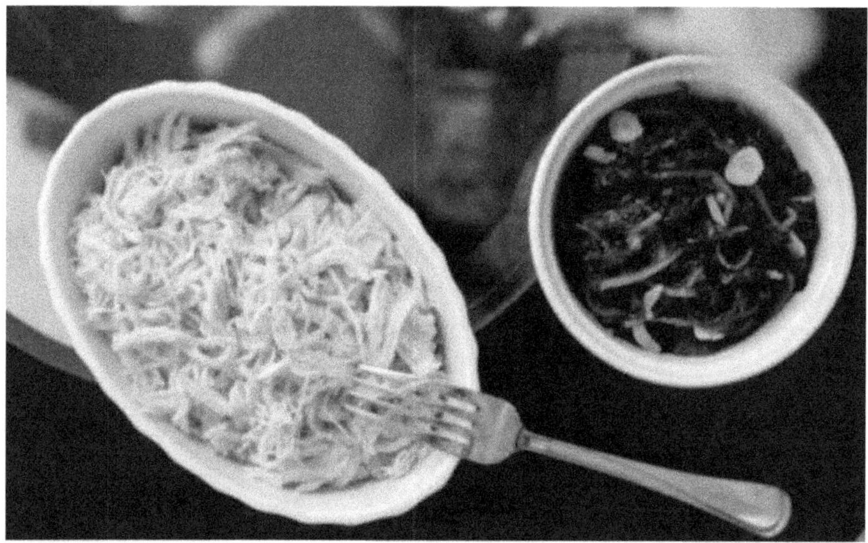

Prep time: 5 minutes
Cook time: 40 minutes
Servings: 4

Ingredients

- 4 well chopped chicken breasts
- Salt to taste
- 10 peeled garlic cloves, diced
- ¼ cup of turmeric ghee

Instructions

1. Put the chicken breasts in the instant pot.
2. Whisk all the ingredients and pour the mixture into the instant pot.
3. Let it cook on high pressure setting for 35 minutes and follow the prompts by the pot to release the pressure.
4. Now, patiently shred the chicken.
5. If desired, add extra ghee and serve.

Nutritional information

Calories: 404
Net carbs: 3g
Proteins: 47g
Fats: 21g

Easy Balsamic Beef Pot Roast

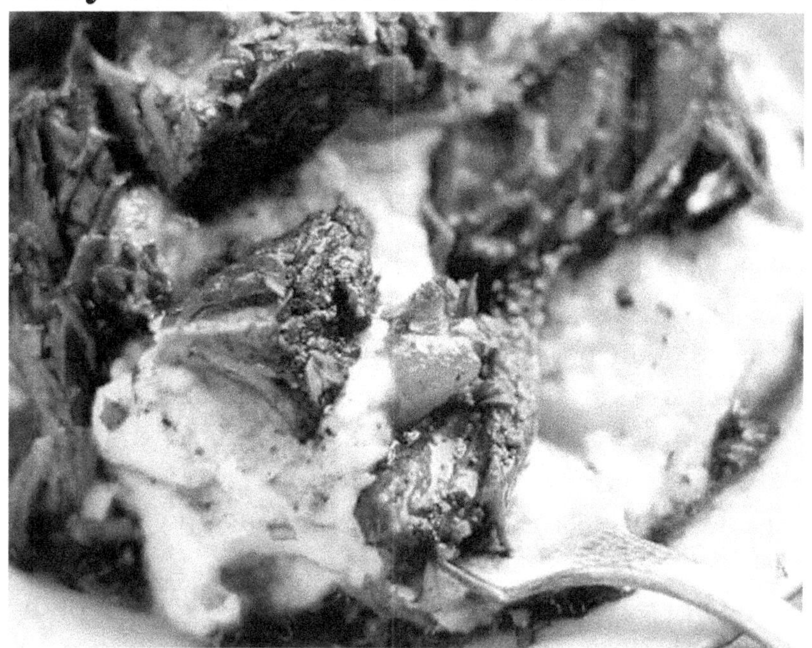

Prep time: 5 minutes
Cook time: 45 minutes
Servings: 4

Ingredients

- 2 cups of water
- ½ cup of finely chopped onion
- ¼ cup of balsamic vinegar
- 1 tsp each ground pepper and garlic powder
- Salt to taste (not more than a tablespoonful, preferably)
- 3 lbs chuck roast, boneless
- 1/4tsp xanthan gum
- Parsley, fresh one for garnishing

Instructions

1. Divide the chuck roast into 2 pieces.
2. Rub the roast with the garlic powder, salt and pepper.
3. Set your instant pot on sauté in order to brown the seasoned roast at both sides.
4. Add in the onion, a cup of water and vinegar. Seal the vent and cover the lid. Set the timer to 35 minutes manual cooking.
5. When it beeps, move the lever to 'venting' in order to release pressure. After releasing the pressure, remove the lid of the pot.
6. Transfer the meat from the Instant pot into a sizable bowl. Carefully break into pieces and remove all unwanted refuse.
7. Reset your instant pot to sauté to boiling the liquid. To reduce, simmer for 10 minutes.
8. Add the xanthan gum and then return the meat into the pot and stir to incorporate well.
9. Turn off the pot. Garnish with freshly chopped parsley and serve delectably on cauliflower puree.

Nutritional information

Calories: 393
Net carbs: 3g
Fats: 28g
Proteins: 30g

Taco Salad

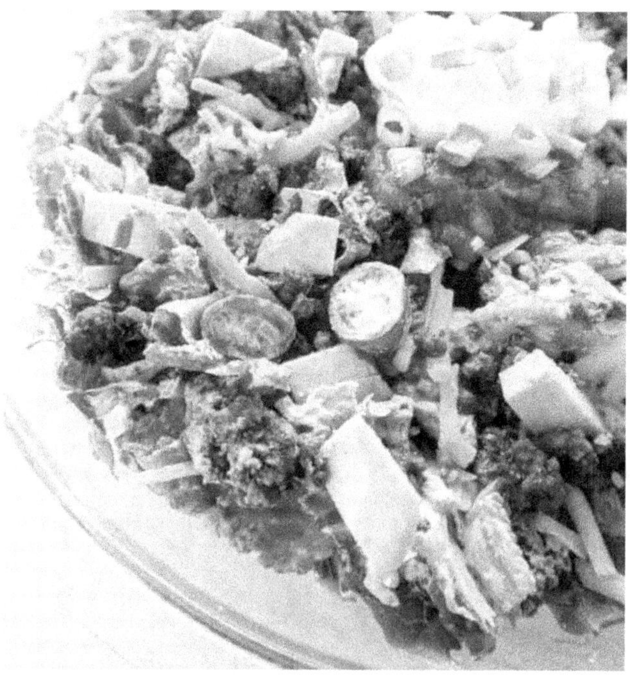

Prep time: 10 minutes
Cook time: 10 minutes
Servings: 6

Ingredients

- 1 lb ground beef
- 1 tsp avocado oil
- 8 oz chopped Romaine lettuce
- 1 tbsp of homemade or store-bought taco seasoning
- 1 1/3 cup of grape tomatoes, divided
- 1/3 cup each salsa and sour cream
- ½ cup of chopped scallions
- 1 cubed avocado, medium size
- ¾ cup of shredded cheddar cheese

Instructions

1. Brown ground beef with onion and garlic.
2. Take off the fat and add in every other ingredient after mixing in a large bowl.
3. Add in taco seasoning and stir until well-incorporated.
4. Put back the ground beef into the pot and stir thoroughly.

Nutritional information

Calories: 332
Net carbs: 5g
Fats: 25g
Protein: 20g

Green Beans Casserole

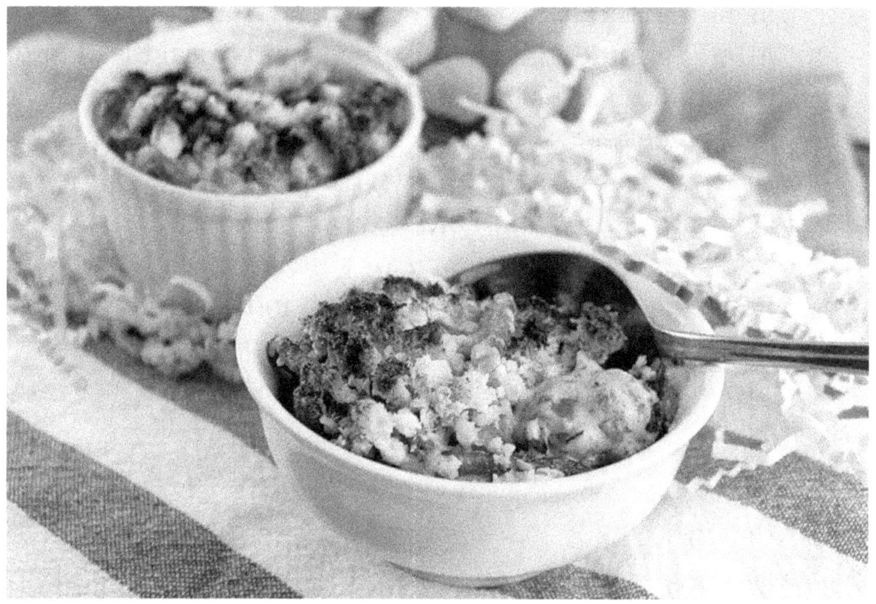

Prep time: 10 minutes
Cook time: 15 minutes
Servings: 4

Ingredients

- 10 oz of green beans
- ½ cup of whipping heavy cream
- Half package of moon cheddar cheese
- Pepper and salt, moderately to taste
- ½ tsp guar gum
- Onion powder, sprinkle
- Bacon, 5 slices

Instructions

1. Finely chop the green onions to make them clean.

2. Next, cut the bacon into tiny pieces and turn your instant pot to sauté. Crush the cheddar in a plastic bag.

3. After 3 minutes, add in the green beans. Seal the vent of the pot and cover it. Use the manual setting to cook for a minute.

4. When it beeps, 'quick release' the pressure.

5. Add in the guar gum and heavy cream. Stir thoroughly to make it incorporate well and thicken quickly.

6. Pour the mixture into ramekins and spread with the onion powder and crushed moon cheese.

7. Broil for 2 minutes and enjoy it hot!

Nutritional information

Calories: 270
Net carbs: 1.8g
Fats: 25.8g
Protein: 7.3g

Creamed Spinach

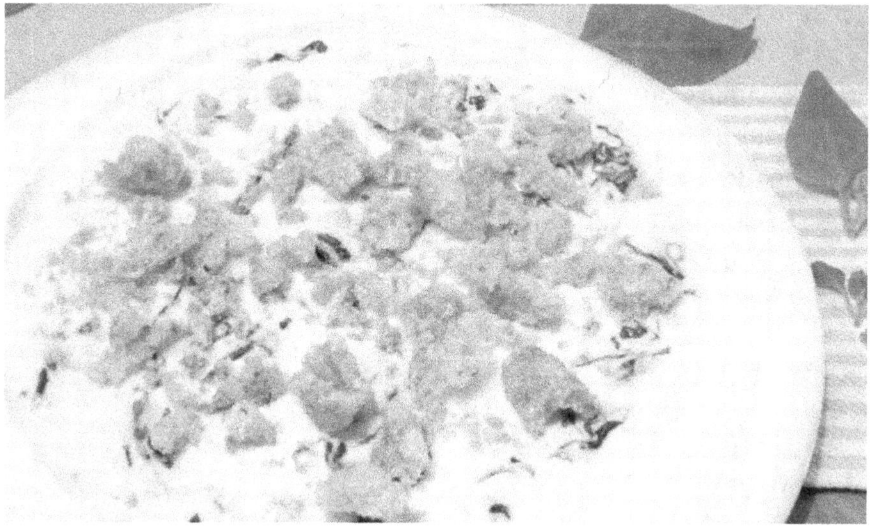

Prep time: 5 minutes
Cook time: 10 minutes
Servings: 8

Ingredients

- 2 minced garlic cloves
- 3 tbsp butter
- 1 tsp of onion powder
- 4 oz cream cheese
- 1 cup of whipping heavy cream
- Pepper and salt to taste
- ½ cup of Romano cheese
- 10 oz of finely chopped spinach, drained and thawed
- 1 tbsp butter

Instructions

1. Pour the 1 tablespoonful of butter into the pot. Add in the Romano cheese, heavy cream and cream cheese.

Turn the pot to medium pressure to melt the cheese and stir well. Add in pepper and salt.

2. After that, transfer the sauce into a large bowl.

3. Turn your instant pot setting to sauté. Add in the 3 tablespoonful of butter, onion powder and garlic.

4. Add in the spinach and stir gently. Cover the pot and cook on low pressure for 5 minutes.

5. Pour the sauce into the pot and stir to incorporate well. Serve it like that!

Nutritional information

Calories: 352
Net carbs: 2g
Fat: 28g
Protein: 13g

Coconut curry chicken

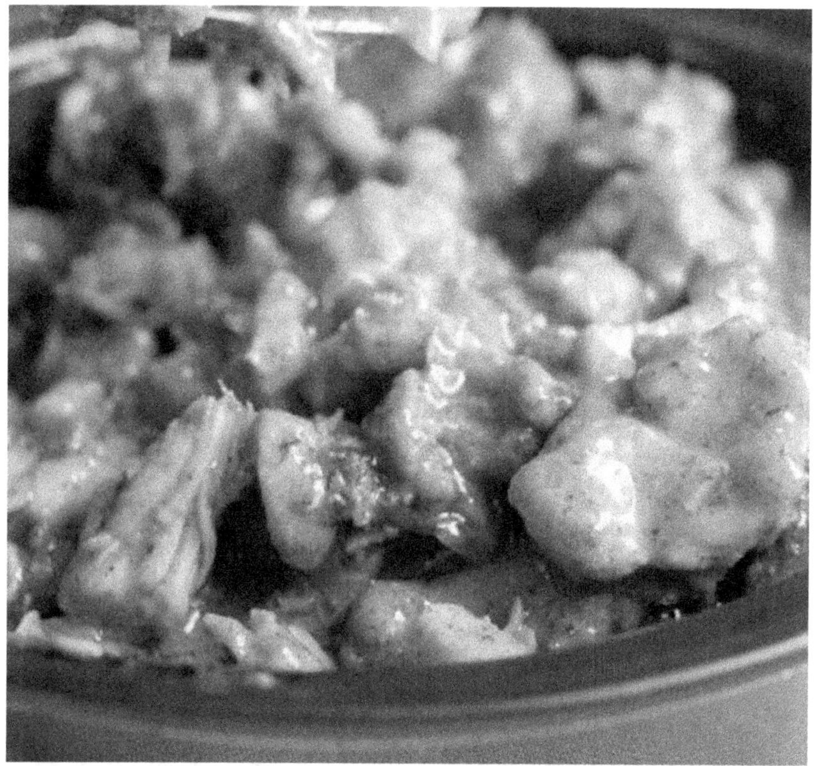

Prep time: 20 minutes
Cook time: 60 minutes
Servings: 5

Ingredients

- 1 cup of chicken broth
- 5 raw chicken thighs, boneless and skinless
- 3 tbsp coconut oil
- 1 tsp ginger, grated
- ¼ medium red onion
- ½ tsp each salt and cinnamon
- 3 garlic cloves
- 1 tbsp curry powder

- 1 can of coconut milk

Instructions

1. Grate ginger and finely chop garlic and onion. Cut the chicken into 1-in cubes.
2. Set your pot on medium-high heat.
3. Add in the chicken and partially cook.
4. Mix cinnamon, curry powder, garlic, ginger and onion together. Pour the mixture on the chicken and cook for 2 minutes.
5. Add in the broth and milk. Stir to combine well.
6. Cook for 40 minutes to achieve needed consistency.

Nutritional information

Calories: 353.8g
Net carbs: 5.6g
Proteins: 26.4g
Fat: 29g

Shepherd's pie

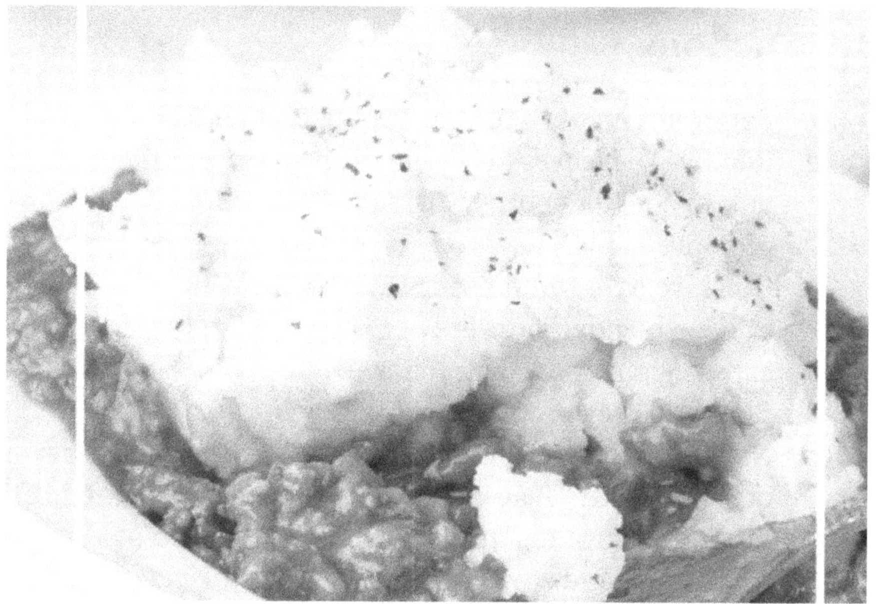

Prep time: 20 minutes
Cook time: 20 minutes
Servings: 12

Ingredients

- 4 oz of cream cheese
- 1 large egg
- A head of cauliflower
- Pepper and salt
- 1 cup of beef broth
- 4 tbsp butter
- 8 oz mushrooms, sliced
- 2 cups of peas, frozen
- Garlic powder
- 1 cup of mozzarella
- 2 lbs ground beef

- 2 cups of well-chopped carrots

Instructions

1. Pour one cup of water into the instant pot.
2. Remove the leaves and stem of the head cauliflower and put inside the pot. Cook for 5 minutes on the high pressure mode.
3. Quick release the pressure and transfer the cauliflower to your blender with the egg, mozzarella, butter, cream cheese, pepper and salt to taste.
4. Blend till they become smooth.
5. Now, take off the steamer rack from the pot and drain off the liquid. Place the garlic powder, ground beef, broth, mushrooms, peas, pepper, carrots and salt in the Instant pot and stir thoroughly.
6. Top it up with the cauliflower mixture, cover the pot and then cook on high pressure for ten minutes.

Nutritional information

Calories: 303
Net carbs: 4.1g
Proteins: 21g
Fat: 21.5g

Citrus Herb Chicken Chorizo

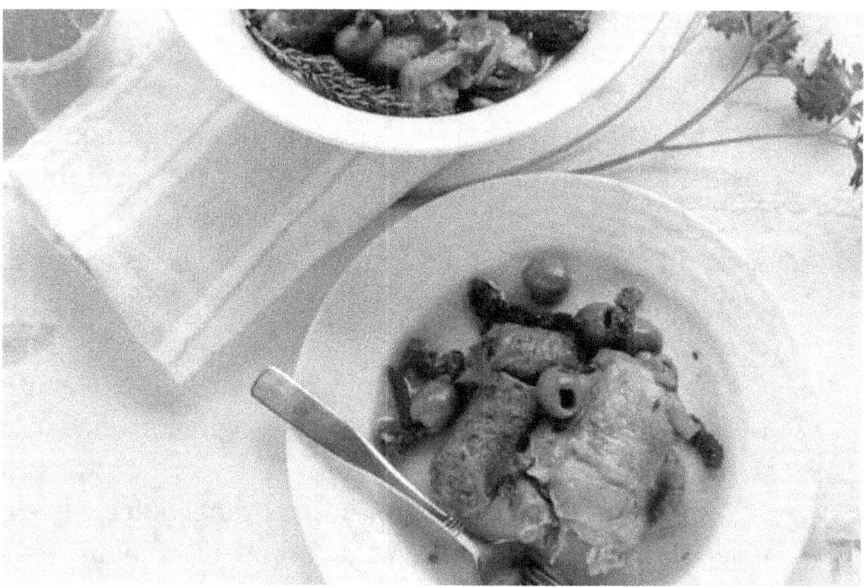

Prep time: 5 minutes
Cook time: 30 minutes
Servings: 4

Ingredients

- 4 chicken thighs, bone-in
- 3 tbsp grass-fed ghee butter
- 1 thickly sliced medium yellow onion
- ½ lb chorizo, with the casing taken off
- 1¼ tbsp divided sea salt
- ½ cup of green olives, pitted
- 1/3 cup of dried tomatoes
- 5 thyme sprigs, stems cut off and leaves weeded
- 1/3 cup of orange juice, just squeezed
- ¾ cup of chicken broth
- 4 minced fresh clove garlic
- Cilantro for garnishing

Instructions

1. Set your instant pot on sauté and pour 2 teaspoonful of fat into the pot.
2. When the fat melts, put the chicken into the pot, put ½ tbsp of sea salt and brown both sides for 5 minutes. After that, take out the chicken into a bowl.
3. Add in the remaining fat, thyme leaves, garlic, remaining salt and onion. Sauté for 5 minutes with occasional stirring.
4. It's time to put the chorizo into the pot. Allow to sauté for another 5 minutes and make sure you stir once in a while.
5. Hit the warm button and add in the orange juice, olives, dried tomatoes and chicken bone broth and stir thoroughly.
6. Submerge the browned chicken in the pot to cook well.
7. Vent the steam and cover the pot. Then, hit the 'poultry' key of your pot. Increase the time to 20 minutes.
8. When it beeps, press the cancel button and quick release the pressure. Carefully uncover the pot.
9. Serve your yummy meal and top with the cilantro.

Nutritional information

Calories: 769
Net carbs: 7g
Protein: 45g
Fat: 50g

Butter chicken curry

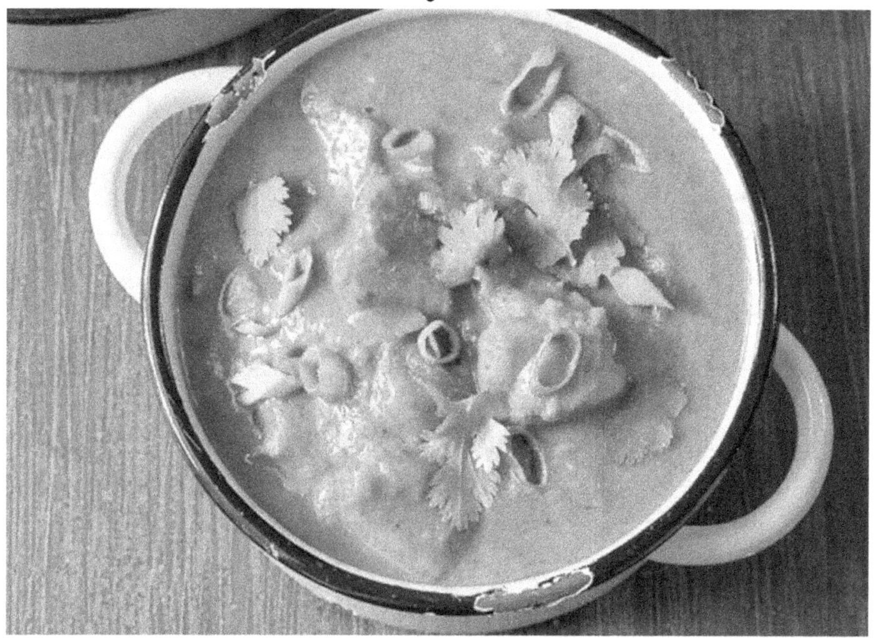

Prep time: 5 minutes
Cook time: 14 minutes
Servings: 8

Ingredients

- 2 lbs chicken thighs, boneless and skinless
- 1 peeled onion, finely chopped
- 4 tbsp ghee
- 1 tbsp curry powder
- 9 minced clove garlic
- 2 tbsp grated ginger
- 1 cup of heavy whipping cream
- Cilantro, well chopped for garnishing
- 15 oz tomato sauce
- Salt to taste
- 1 tsp smoked paprika

- 2 tbsp garam masala

Instructions

1. Set your instant pot on sauté and add in butter. Also place garlic, onion, ginger and every other spice in the pot. Sauté for 5 minutes with occasional stirring. Switch off the pot when they become soft.
2. Add in tomato sauce and chicken thighs. Vent the seal and cover the pot. Cook on high pressure for 7 minutes and immediately after it beeps, perform quick release to get rid of the steam pressure.
3. After that, uncover the pot and put the heavy whipping cream in it. Reset your pot on sauté and simmer for about 2 minutes so as to make the sauce thick.
4. Garnish with the freshly chopped cilantro and serve your yummy meal. It is so delicious with basmati rice.

Nutritional information

Calories: 351
Net carbs: 5.3g
Proteins: 33g
Fat: 21g

Creamy chicken bacon chowder

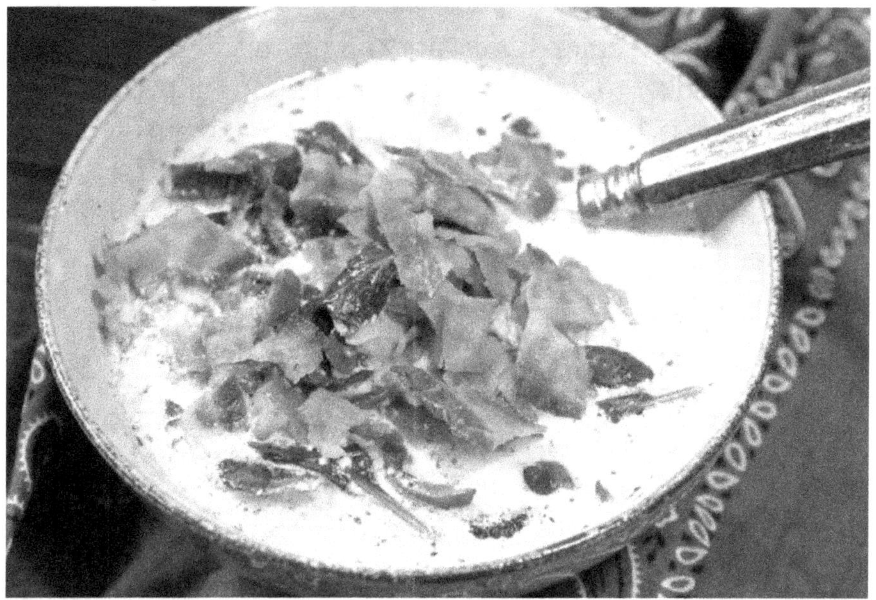

Prep time: 10 minutes
Cook time: 30 minutes
Servings: 5

Ingredients

- 6 chicken thighs, boneless and skinless
- 4 tsp minced garlic cloves
- 4 tbsp butter
- Pepper and salt, moderately to taste
- 1 tsp thyme
- 1 finely chopped onion
- 6 oz mushrooms, sliced
- 8 oz full fat cream cheese
- 1 cup of heavy cream
- 3 cups of chicken broth
- 2 cups of spinach, fresh
- 1 lb chopped cooked bacon

Instructions

1. Add in the chicken mixture and broth to the pot and set the cooker to 'soup'. Let it cook for 30 minutes.
2. When it beeps, stir thoroughly and add in the heavy cream and fresh spinach.
3. Cover the pot and allow it cook for another 10 minutes for spinach to wilt.
4. Garnish with cooked bacon and serve.

Nutritional information

Calories: 201
Net carbs: 3g
Proteins: 5.1g
Fat: 19.1g

Meatballs and sauce

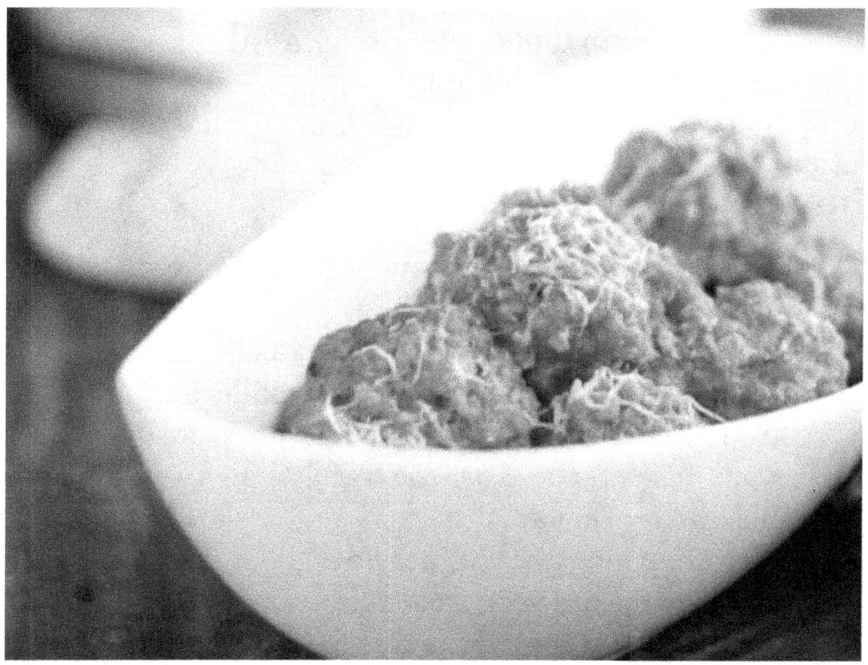

Prep time: 10 minutes
Cook time: 20 minutes
Servings: 5

Ingredients

- 1 ½ lbs ground beef
- 2 large eggs
- 1/3 cup of warm water
- ¼ tsp each garlic powder and black pepper
- 1 tsp dried onion flakes
- ¼ tsp of oregano, dried
- 1 tbsp Kosher salt
- ½ cup of almond flour
- ¾ cup of parmesan cheese, grated
- 2 tbsp of freshly chopped parsley

For meatballs

- 3 cups of *easy keto marinara sauce* (other sugar-free sauces can be used as well)
- 1 tsp olive oil

Instructions

1. Use hands to thoroughly mix meatball ingredients in a medium-sized bowl.
2. Make it into about 15 two-inch meatballs.
3. Add in the olive oil into the bottom of the instant pot.
4. You can brown them by turning on the sauté function of your instant pot. Turn on regular intervals for both sides to brown well.
5. Lay them in the pot, leaving about an inch space between the browned meatballs.
6. Evenly spread the marinara sauce on the 2 meatballs.
7. Seal pot and switch to manual cooking.
8. Hit the low pressure button and cook for 10 minutes.
9. Once it beeps, switch the valve of the instant pot to vent and let steam dissipate fully.
10. Uncover the pot and serve your healthy meatballs on spaghetti squash.

Nutritional information

Calories: 455
Net carbs: 5g
Protein: 34g
Fat: 33g

Mississippi pot roast

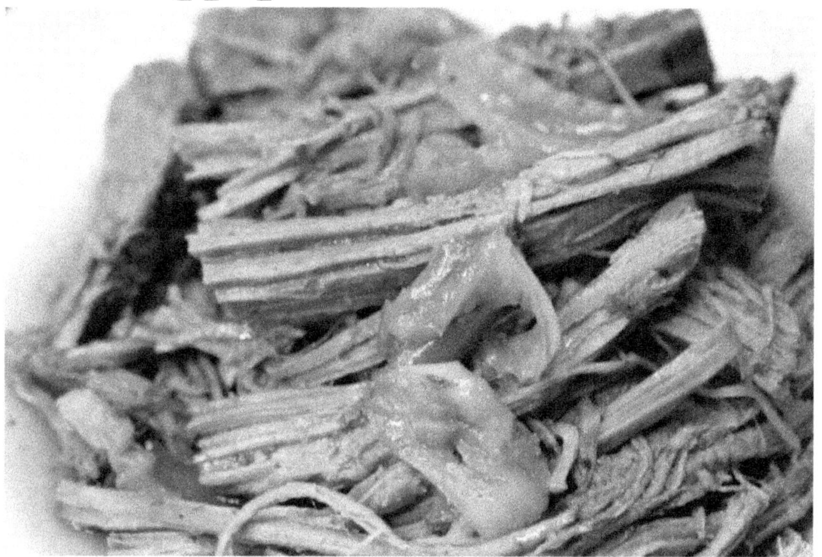

Prep time: 10 minutes

Cook time: 1hr 30 minutes

Servings: 6

Ingredients

- ½ cup of water
- ½ cup of butter
- 1 packet ranch seasoning mix
- ½ jar peppercinis (the juice inclusive)
- 1¾ lbs of roast

Ingredients

1. Put the roast in the instant pot.
2. Spray the packet of ranch seasoning on the roast.
3. Add butter and peppercinis.

4. Add some water on the roast.

5. Seal the vent and cover the pot. Press the manual cooking button and set time to 90 minutes.

6. When it beeps, gently shred and it's time for serving.

Nutritional information

Calories: 548
Net carb: 2g
Fat: 34.2g
Protein: 40g

Parmesan Garlic Artichokes

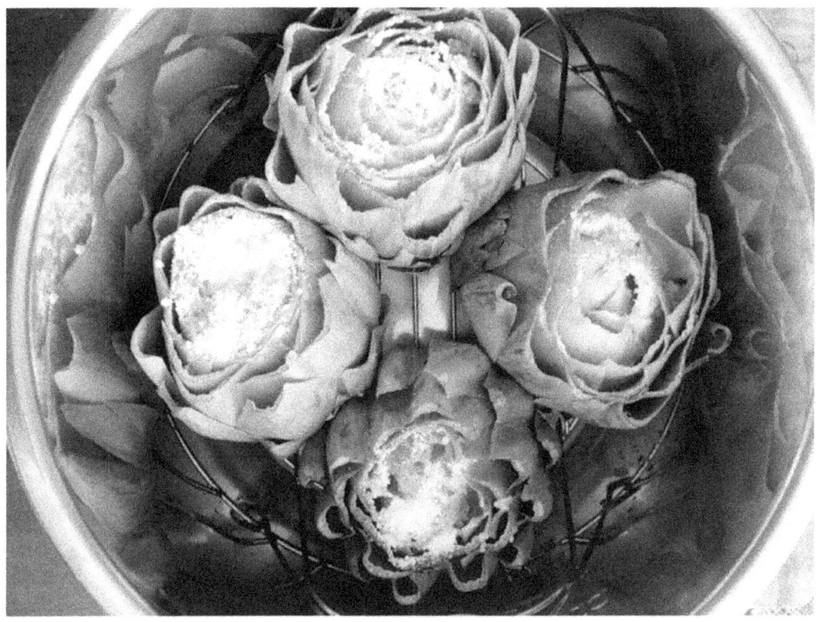

Prep time: 10 minutes
Cook time: 7 minutes
Servings: 8

Ingredients

- 2 tsp garlic, minced
- 4 pieces of artichokes
- 4 tsp olive oil
- 1/2 cup chicken broth (you can also use water instead)
- ¼ cup of grated parmesan cheese or shredded one

Instructions

1. Clean and chop artichokes, ridding it of its head, steam and outer leaves.
2. Sprinkle each of the 4 artichokes with ½ teaspoon of garlic and top with a teaspoonful of olive oil.

3. Spray the artichokes with 4 tablespoonful of parmesan cheese.
4. Get place the artichokes in the pot through basket insert. You may now add the chicken broth or use water instead of the broth.
5. Seal the valve of the pot, hit the 'steam' button and cook for 10 minutes.
6. Once it beeps, quick release the pressure. And your delicious healthy meal is ready!

Nutritional information

Calories: 150
Net carbs 5g
Protein: 11g
Fat: 10g

Ketogenic soups

Chicken Enchilada Soup

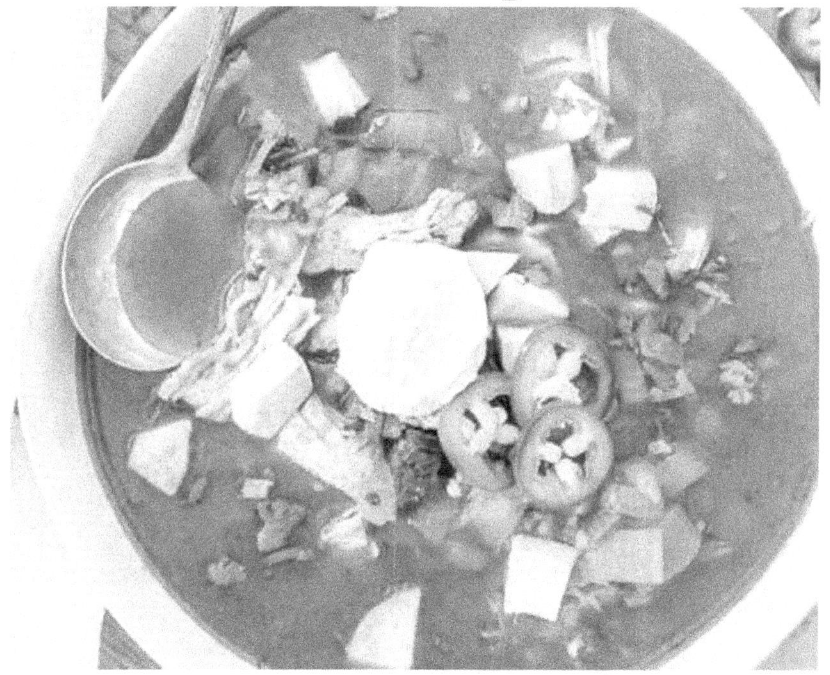

Preparation time: 10 minutes
Cook time: 30 minutes
Servings: 4

Ingredients

- 1 tbsp olive oil
- 3 minced garlic cloves
- 1 large diced bell pepper
- 1 minced jalapeno
- 8 oz tomato sauce, sugar-free
- 1 tbsp each chili and garlic powder
- 2 tbsp cumin, ground
- 1 tbsp white vinegar and onion powder

- 1 lb chicken breasts
- 3 cups of chicken broth
- Sea salt to taste

Instructions

1. Set the instant pot to sauté and then pour the olive oil into it.
2. Immediately, add the garlic, onion, jalapeno and bell peppers and cook for minutes.
3. Mix other ingredients very well and then pour it into the cooker.
4. It's time to add your chicken and broth before stirring.
5. Cover the pot and reset it to high manual mode for 20 minutes before releasing the vent valve.
6. Use a knife and fork to shred your chicken and after that, return it into the pot.
7. It's ready and you may top it with avocado or sour cream. And it's ready to be devoured!

Nutritional information

Calories: 268
Net carbs: 8g
Total fat: 24g
Protein: 28g
Fiber:4g

Chili soup

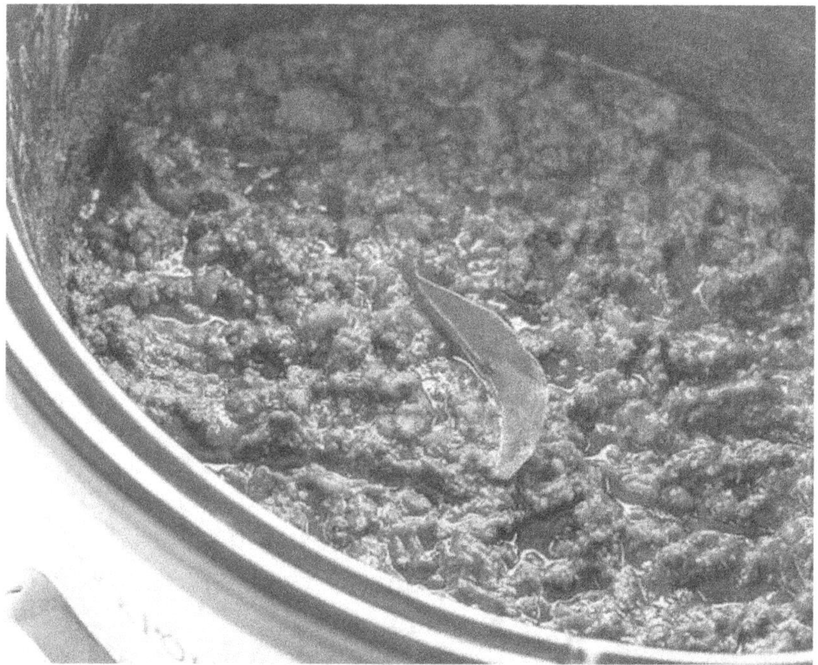

Prep time: 15 minutes
Cook time: 1 hour 15 minutes
Servings: 10

Ingredients

- 2 ½ beef, ground
- 1 small onion, finely chopped
- 8 minced garlic cloves
- Tomato paste and green chiles (1 each)
- ¼ cup of chili powder
- 2 tbsp sauce
- 2 cans diced tomatoes
- 1 tbsp oregano, dried
- 2 tbsp sea salt
- 1 tbsp black pepper

Instructions

1. Select the sauté setting of your pressure cooker without the lid.
2. Pour the finely chopped onion into the pot and allow leave it for 7 minutes to translucent. However, if you prefer the caramelized form, allow it to cook for 20 minutes.
3. You can now put the garlic and allow 1 minute more for cooking.
4. Now, it's time to add your beef and allow cooking for 10 minutes. During this time, you should get a spatula to break it and make the beef brown.
5. Add every other ingredient and broth. Gently stir till everything becomes well-combined and yummy!
6. It's time for pressure cooking! Cover the pot and leave it on a high mode for 40 minutes.
7. Patiently wait for it to be released naturally and without hesitation, it's time for serving!

Nutritional Information

Calories: 306
Net carbs: 5g
Protein: 13g
Fat: 18g
Fiber: 3g

Cabbage soup

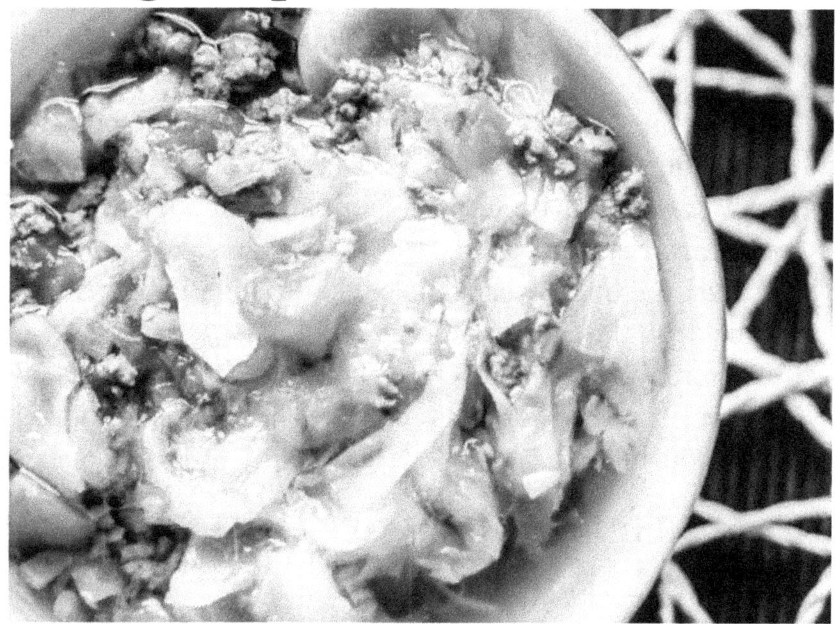

Preparation time: 5 minutes
Cook time: 40 minutes
Servings: 10

Ingredients

- 2 lbs ground beef
- ½ diced onion
- 1 tbsp ground cumin
- 1 large cabbage, finally chopped
- Water (about 4 cups)
- Pepper and salt (moderately to taste)
- 1 minced garlic clove
- Diced tomatoes (10 oz) and 1 can of green chilies

Instructions

1. Set your instant pot on medium to brown the ground beef.
2. Pour the diced onion inside it until it becomes translucent.
3. Now, add every other ingredient and stir very well until they are well combined.
4. Adjust the heat level of the cooker to high mode so as to quickly make the ingredients mix up.
5. Then, cover it and reset the heat level to medium-low. Leave it for about 45 minutes and your soup is deliciously ready!

Nutritional information

Saturated fat: 7g
Total fat: 18g
Calories: 261
Net carbs: 4g
Protein: 15g

Summer vegetable soup

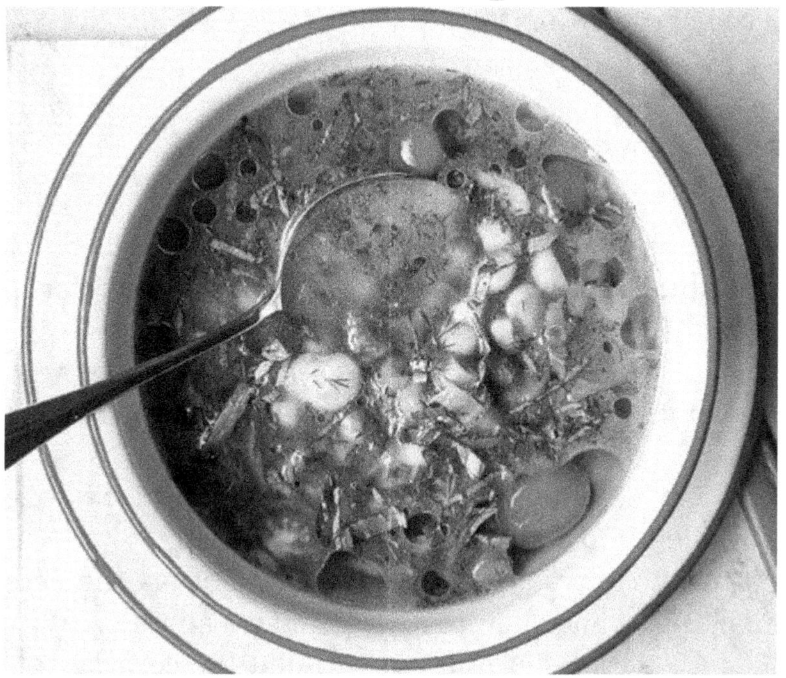

Prep time: 50 minutes
Cooking time: 60 minutes

Servings: 5

Ingredients

- 1 tsp ground pepper
- 3 tbsp olive oil
- 1 large yellow onion, well chopped and peeled
- 2 qt homemade chicken stock
- 1 tbsp fine turmeric
- Salt to taste
- 2 garlic, minced
- ¼lb trimmed beans
- ½ cup of peas with another ½ cup of peeled lima beans

- 1 tbsp Lime juice
- 1 cup of cherry tomatoes
- ¾ tbsp mixed dill, chives and parsley
- ½ cup of corn kernels

Instructions

1. In your instant pot, heat the extra-virgin olive oil.
2. Add the minced garlic and allow it to cook for 2 minutes.
3. You can now add your finely chopped onions with moderate salt and then allow it to cook for about 5 minutes.
4. You may now add the turmeric and chicken stock while you allow it to boil for about 30 minutes.
5. At this point, you can add peeled lima beans and peas into the pot and allow to boil for about a minute.
6. Reduce the heat of the pot and add the corn kernels while you leave it to boil for 3 minutes.
7. Add seasoning, pepper and salt and then, it is ready to be served!

Nutritional information

Calories: 210
Protein: 13g
Fats: 20g
Net carbs: 2g

Hamburger stew

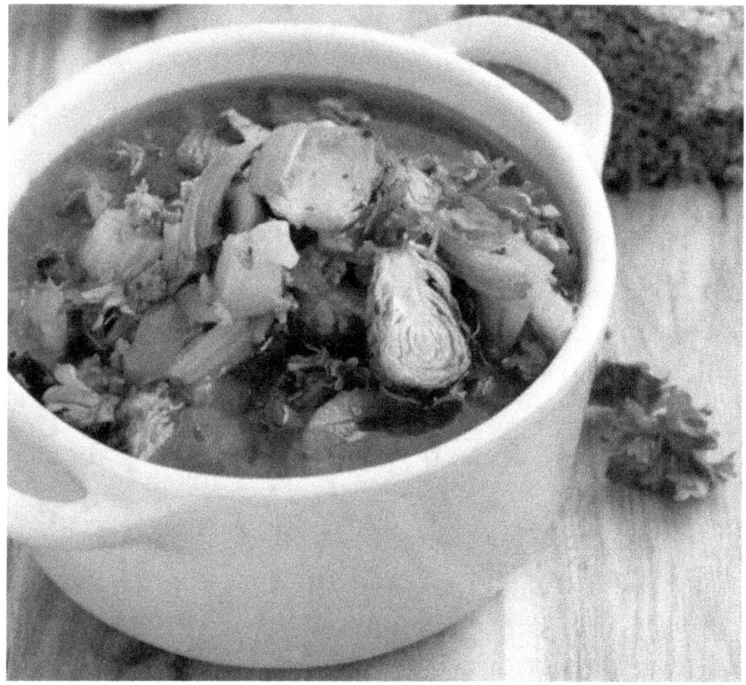

Prep time: 30 minutes
Cooking time: 40 minutes
Servings: 6

Ingredients

- 1 well sliced red onion
- 9 finely chopped mushrooms
- 1 sliced yellow bell pepper
- 18 Brussels sprouts
- Moderate amount of palm oil (about ¼ of a cup)
- Ground pepper and rock salt in desired but advisably low quantity
- 1 lb of grass-fed beef
- 3 well minced garlic
- 6 sticks of celery

- Beef stock (4 cups and the fat inclusive)
- 1 tbsp tomato paste, organic
- 1 bay leaf with 1 tbsp of oregano, dried
- ¼ cup finely chopped parsley
- Chili powder and cayenne pepper to taste

Instructions

1. Allow your pressure cooker to sauté.
2. You can now pout the mushroom, pepper, salt, palm oil and Brussels sprouts into the instant pot.
3. Allow the veggies to roast for about 25 minutes.
4. Add your beef, celery and garlic and cook for about 5 minutes.
5. Add spices, paste and tomatoes, reducing the heat level of the cooker to minimum and allow it to simmer for 17 minutes.
6. Gently stir everything together and it's ready to be served!

Nutritional Information (per serving)

Calories: 478
Fats: 34.5g
Protein: 27g
Net carbs: 10g
Saturated fats: 14.7g

Creamy Chicken Soup

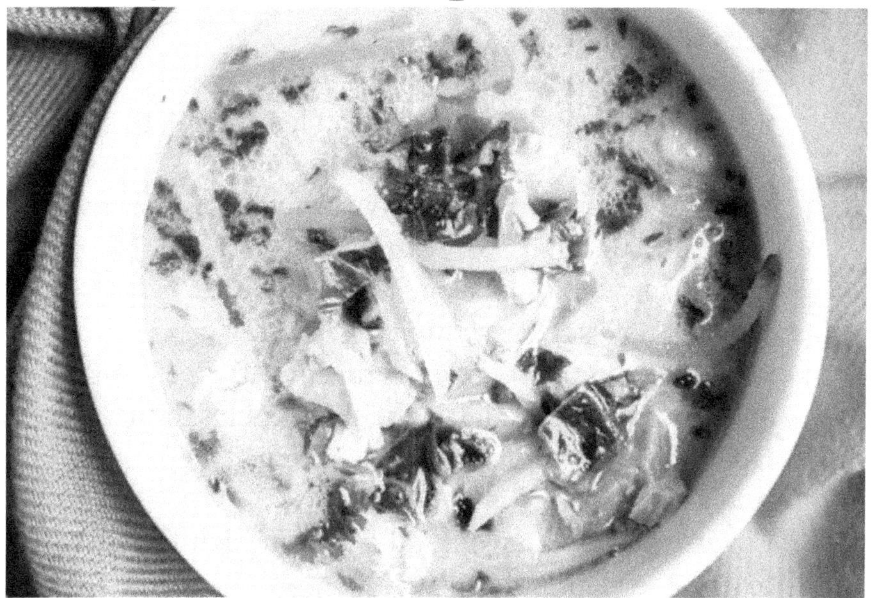

Prep time: 10 minutes
Cooking time: 10 minutes
Servings: 4

Ingredients

- 1 large diced onion
- 1 tbsp avocado oil
- 1 lb chicken thighs, boneless and skinless
- ¾ divided bone broth
- 1 tbsp each salt, dried thyme and garlic powder
- 1 diced avocado
- 1 can coconut milk, full fat
- Juice, one lemon
- 1 tbsp fish sauce
- 1 bag blend

Instructions

1. Let your instant pot sauté.
2. Then, pour your avocado oil into the cooker. You can now add the onion and garlic and leave them to cook for 7 minutes.
3. In order to allow the chicken brown, gently move the garlic and onion aside. Let the chicken touch bottom of the cooker while you leave it for 6 minutes.
4. You can now stir everything together.
5. Add seasoning and bone broth. After this, close the pot and leave for it to boil for about 5 minutes at high level.
6. Open the cover and shred the chicken.
7. Add the milk, juice and blend.
8. Cover the cooker again and set it on high level to cook for another 2 minutes.
9. Now, you can manually release the cooker, stir gently and it's ready to be served!
10. You may garnish it with diced avocado.

Nutritional Information

Saturated fats: 13g
Protein: 18g
Total fat: 25g
Calories: 307

Chicken Tortilla Soup

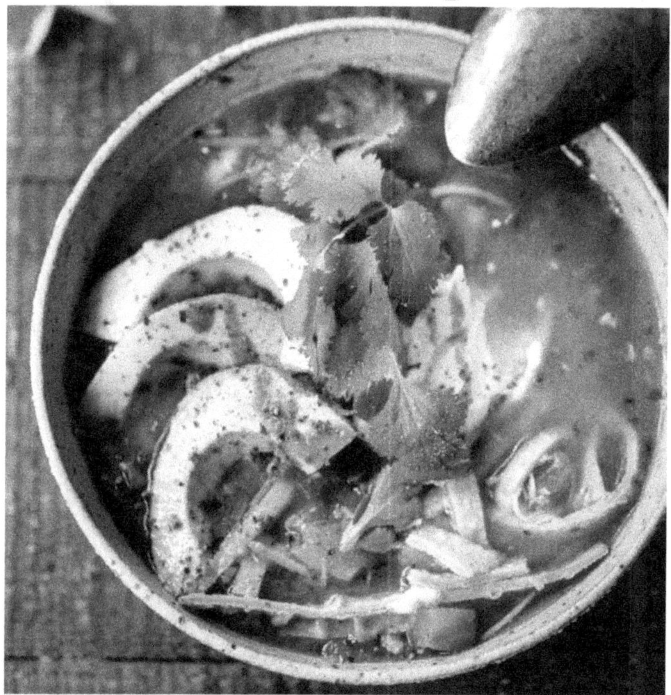

Prep time: 10 minutes
Cooking time: 20 minutes
Servings: 6

Ingredients

- 2 chicken breasts, boneless and skinless
- 1 can of low-sodium beans, black
- 1 cup kernel corn
- 1 tbsp each chilis and tomatoes, diced
- Chicken broth, 32 oz low in sodium
- lemon juice to taste
- 1 finely chopped small onion
- 1 tbsp flavor
- 3 garlic cloves, peeled and chopped
- ½ cup tomato paste, seasoning

- 2 tbsp cilantro
- Tortilla strips (½ cup)
- Shredded cheese (½ cup)

Instructions

1. Let your instant pot sauté.
2. Pour the garlic and chopped onions into the pot and allow cooking for about 3 minutes.
3. After that, add in the chicken breast, broth, seasoning, tomato paste and flavor.
4. Cover the lid and allow cooking for 10 minutes with the cooker being on high mode.
5. Let the steam be naturally released for 10 minutes (avoid performing quick release).
6. Uncover the pot and shred the chicken with a knife.
7. Add in the lemon juice, beans and corn and then, stir gently to mix.
8. Allow 4 minutes cooking for all the added ingredients to soften at the same rate.
9. Now, you can serve and top the soup with cheese, cilantro and tortilla strips.

Nutritional Information

Calories: 339
Protein: 13g
Net carbs: 1.5g
Fat: 30g

Chicken Noodle Soup

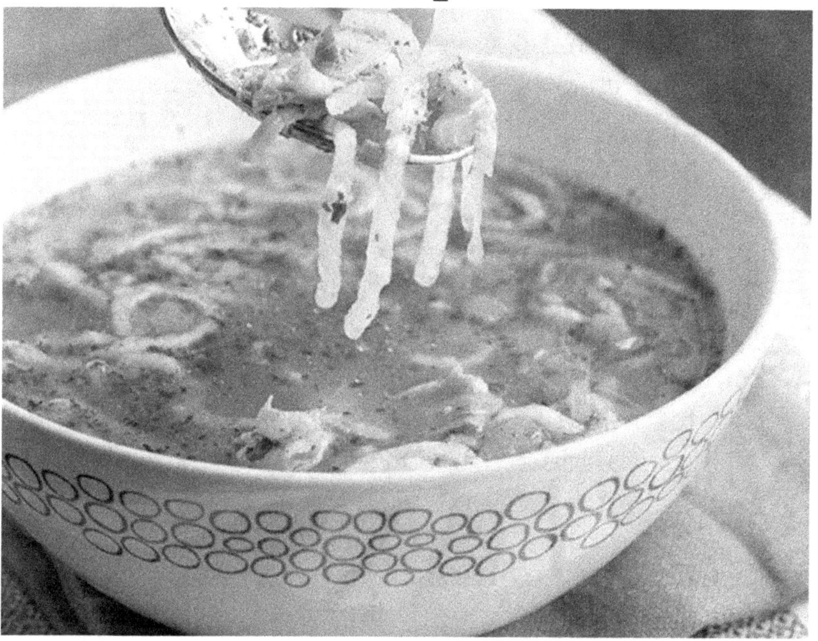

Prep time: 10 minutes
Cook time: 15 minutes
Servings: 4

Ingredients

- 2 tbsp of coconut oil
- 1 lb chicken thighs, boneless and skinless
- 1 cup of celery, diced
- 2 daikon noodles, spiralized or veggies peelers
- ½ tsp ground pepper
- ½ cup each basil and oregano, both dried
- 1 cup of diced carrots and sea salt
- 1 cup carrots and celery, diced
- 6 finely chopped green onions
- Chicken stocks, 6 cups and a cup of diced celery

Instructions

1. Sauté the instant pot.
2. Place the chicken thighs and oil in the bowl of the cooker.
3. Then, cook the chicken for 10 minutes.
4. After that, you can shred the chicken with fork and knife.
5. Add onions, carrots and celery and cook for 2 minutes.
6. Now, every other ingredient can delectably go in.
7. Put the lid on it and set the cooker on high mode for 15 minutes for the soup to properly cook.
8. It's time to add the noodles or vegetable peelers and then, serving time!

Nutritional information

Calories: 260
Net carbs: 2g
Fat: 28g
Protein: 14g

Goulash Soup

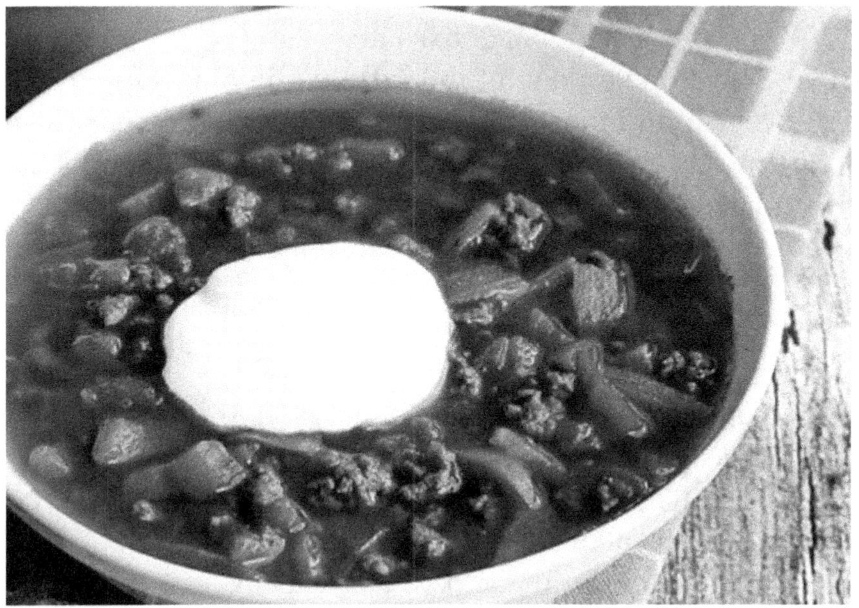

Prep time:
Cook time:
Servings: 7

Ingredients

- 2 lbs ground beef (90% lean)
- 3 tbsp olive oil
- 1 bell pepper
- 1 large finely chopped onion
- 1 garlic, minced
- Sweet and hot Hungarian paprika (2 tablespoon and ½ respectively)
- Beef stock, 4 cups of homemade or beef broth of 3 cans
- 2 cans diced tomatoes

Instructions

1. Set your instant pot onto sauté.
2. Pour 2 tablespoon of the extra virgin olive oil into the cooker and then quickly break the beef and pour them into the pot to cook. While cooking, you can also break them with turner.
3. After the beef becomes brown, you can remove it into a bowl.
4. Then, it's time to cook the meats; while cooking, you should cut them into strips.
5. Add in the onion, red pepper and the remaining 1 tablespoonful of olive oil and cook for 4 minutes.
6. Now, it's time to add the paprika (sweet and hot) and garlic and allow 3 minutes cooking.
7. Add in the broth or beef stock along with the diced tomatoes. Cover the pot and set it to 'soup' with 15 minutes of cooking time.
8. When it's done, give room for manual releasing of pressure for some minutes before using the quick release to finish it up.
9. And it's simply ready to be served! If it's your wish, with a sour cream.

Nutritional information

Calories: 254
Protein: 15g
Net carbs: 3g
Fat: 21g

Cauliflower Soup

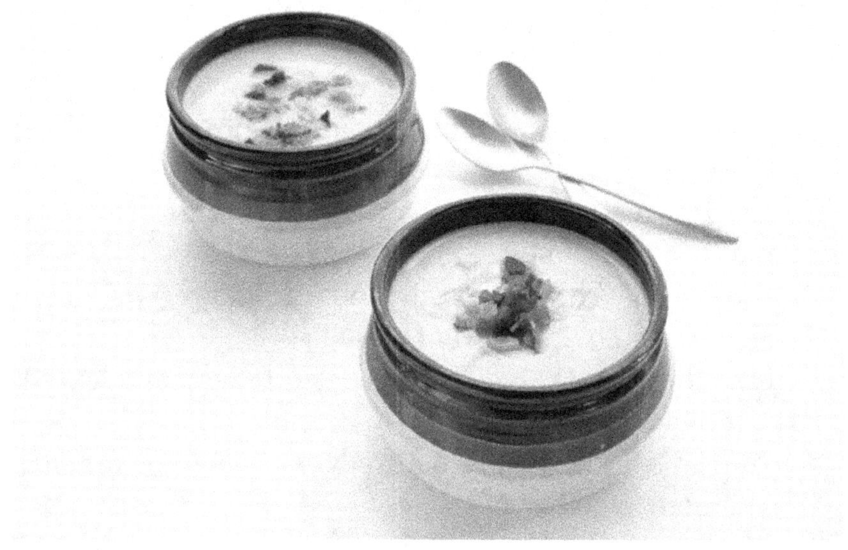

Prep time: 15 minutes
Cooking time: 25 minutes
Servings: 6

Ingredients

- ½ cup small onions
- 1 chopped stalk celery
- 2 minced garlic cloves
- 1 large green onion
- 1½ cups of divided cheddar
- ¾ cup sour cream
- 1 head of cauliflower, florets
- 3 cups chicken broth
- Moderate pepper and salt to taste

Instructions

1. Set your instant pot onto the sauté function.
2. Then, pour the bacon into the pot and keep stirring until crisp.
3. While leaving the fat in the pot, remove the crisped bacon into a plate.
4. Add in every other ingredient and cook for 4 minutes and then you can turn down the sauté.
5. Add in the chicken broth and cauliflower and then cover the pot with the vent sealed.
6. Turn the control mode of the cooker to high and leave it to cook for 5 minutes.
7. After this, let it release naturally for some few minutes and then open the vent.
8. Stir the sour cream and cheese thoroughly until they are well-mixed with other ingredients.
9. After blending, you can delectably top your soup with green onion, leftover cheese and the bacon.

Nutritional information

Calories: 325
Protein: 14g
Net carbs: 7g
Fat: 24g

Ketogenic Sauces

Peanut Sauce

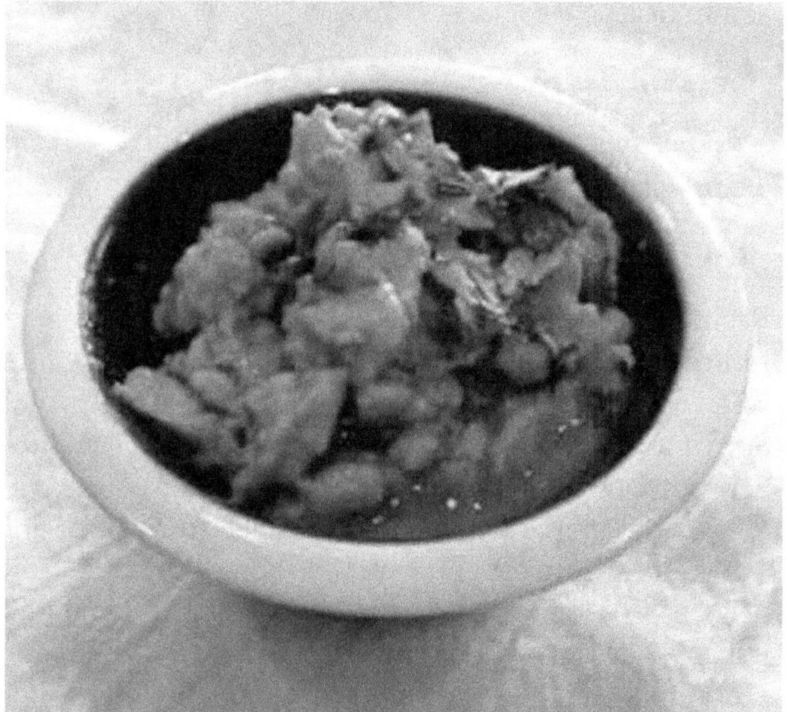

Prep time: 5 minutes
Cook time: 15 minutes
Servings: 4

Ingredients

- 2 tsp coconut oil
- 2 garlic cloves
- 1 lb ground chicken
- 1 tsp ginger, well minced

For the sauce

- ½ cup of hot water
- ¼ cup creamy peanut butter

- 1 tsp each soy sauce and sriracha sauce
- 2 tbsp of chile sauce
- Lime juice to taste
- Salt to taste

Ingredients for garnish

- 3 tbsp peanuts, crushed
- 6 tsp well chopped cilantro

Instructions

1. Begin by heating the coconut oil in a saucepan.
2. In order to fragrance the coconut oil, add in the garlic when it begins to smoke.
3. Stir continuously for about a minute.
4. Set your instant pot on sauté, then add in the chicken.
5. Mix all the ingredients and pour in the half cup of hot water and stir thoroughly until it becomes smooth.
6. After setting your pot on the 'low pressure', pour the mixed sauce on the ground chicken and then stir everything together.
7. Now, cover the pot for it to simmer and to allow the sauce become thick.
8. You should uncover it after 5 minutes, then add the cilantro and peanuts as garnish. Cilantro makes the sauce deliciously tasty.
9. It's time to serve and I bet you, it will be yummy!

Nutritional information

Calories: 289
Net carbs: 5g
Fat: 24g
Protein: 17g

Barbeque Chicken

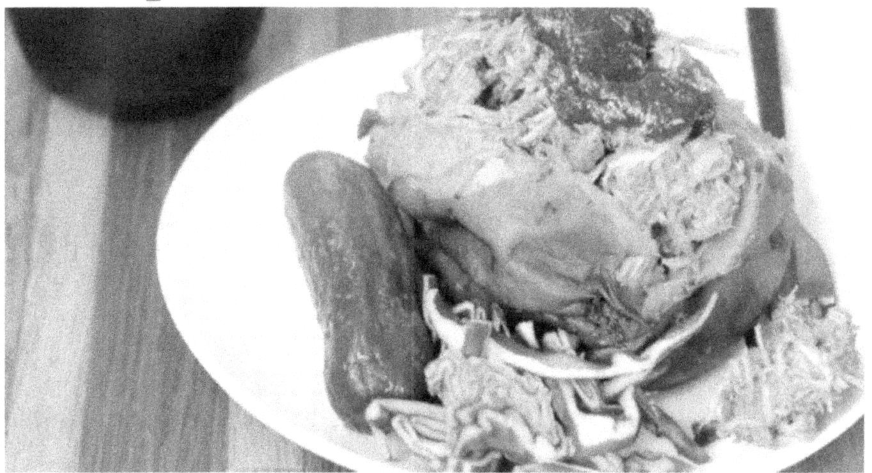

Prep time: 5 minutes
Cook time: 24 minutes
Servings: 5

Ingredients

- 3 lbs chicken breasts, boneless and skinless or an organic chicken thigh
- 7 oz tomato paste, organic
- ¼ cup of cider vinegar
- Stevia extract, 2 dunks
- ¾ cup of bone broth

For the sauce

- 2 tbsp soy sauce, naturally fermented
- 2 tsp of blackstrap molasses, unsulphured
- 1 tbsp each of onion powder and natural liquid smoke
- 2 tsp each organic flavor and garlic powder
- 2 tsp salt and mustard
- 1 tsp chipotle powder
- ½ tsp allspice

Instructions

1. Get a clean bowl and mix all the ingredients properly until they become very smooth.
2. Drop your chicken breasts in the pot and pour the mixed ingredients on it.
3. Seal the vent and cover the pot.
4. Hit the 'poultry' setting of your pot and with a maximum of 24 minutes to cook.
5. After that, release the pressure naturally.
6. Use things to remove the chicken from the pot.
7. Then, get a fork and a knife to shred the chicken or use a stand mixer to get it done.

Nutritional information

Calories: 307
Protein: 7g
Net carbs: 3g
Fat: 18g

Beef Curry

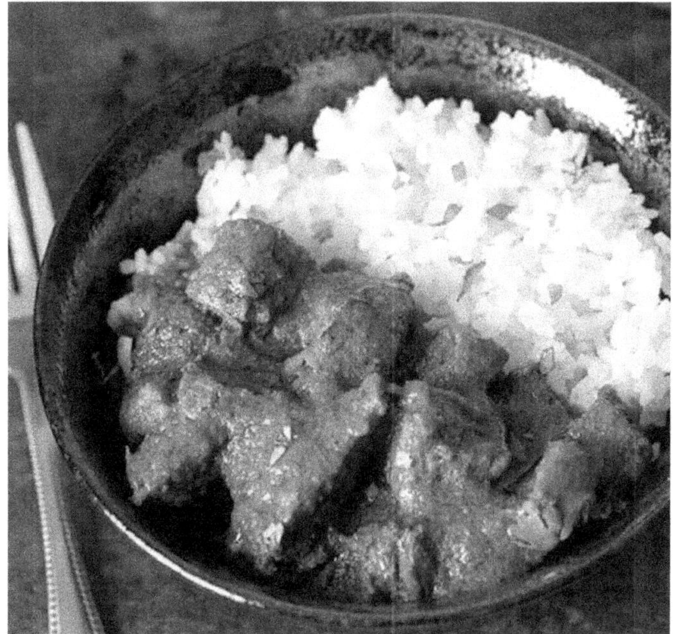

Prep time: 5 minutes
Cook time: 30 minutes
Servings: 4

Ingredients

- 1 finely chopped onion
- 2 sliced tomatoes
- 4 chopped garlic cloves
- ½ cup of cilantro
- 1 lb beef roast

For the sauce

- Seasoning and salt moderately to taste
- ½ tbsp. cayenne pepper
- 1 tsp each garam Masala and ground cumin
- 1/3 tsp coriander

Instructions

1. Place the tomatoes, onions, garlic and cilantro in a blender jar and process it until they turn to a puree.
2. Add in the masala, pepper, salt, cumin and coriander and process further for some few more minutes.
3. Place the beef in the liner of the pot and pour the mixed ingredients on it.
4. Cover the instant pot and allow it cook for 20 minutes.
5. Let the pressure release naturally for 10 minutes.
6. Uncover the pot and stir gently. It's ready to be served!

Nutritional information

Calories: 400
Net carbs: 6g
Protein: 15g
Fat: 30g

Ribs with White Barbecue Sauce

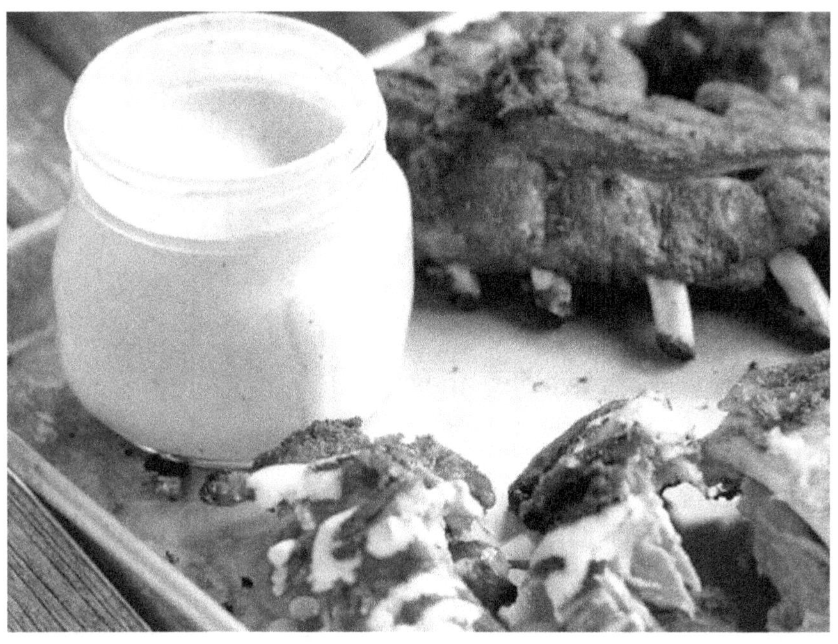

Prep time: 10 minutes

Cook time: 2hrs 50 minutes

Servings: 5

Ingredients

For ribs

- 1 cup of water
- 2 tsp liquid smoke
- ¼ cup of apple cider vinegar
- 3 lbs ribs, baby back

For the rub

- ½ tbsp each garlic and onion powders
- ½ tsp each black and cayenne peppers

- ½ tsp of dried mustard
- 1 tsp salt
- ½ tsp cumin
- ½ tbsp of chili powder
- 1 tbsp of paprika

For the sauce

- 1½ cup of mayonnaise
- ¼ cup of apple cider vinegar
- 1 tsp salt
- 1 tsp minced garlic
- 2 tsp horseradish, prepared
- 2 tbsp of swerve
- 1 tsp black pepper
- 1 tsp Dijon mustard

Instructions

1. Pour all the ingredients for the rub in a bowl and mix properly. Then, rinse the ribs with water and dry them.
2. Take off the silver skin from the ribs.
3. Use the spice rub to season the ribs. Ensure you rub all the sides well so that they become well-coated.
4. Now, add in the water, liquid smoke and vinegar into the bowl of instant pot and place the trivet on it. Add in the seasoned ribs.
5. Seal the vent and cover the pot. Let it cook for 35 minutes on Manual High setting. When it beeps, let it naturally release pressure.

6. Mix the sauce ingredients in a bowl. Use a blender to blend the ingredients. Put sauce in fridge for more than 2 hours so as to allow flavor combine properly.

7. After preheating the grill to 450°F degrees, grill each side of the ribs for 6 minutes until it becomes crispy.

8. Enjoy the ribs with the sauce!

Nutritional information

Calories: 645.83

Net carbs: 2.38g

Protein: 57g

Fat: 43g

Tzatziki Sauce

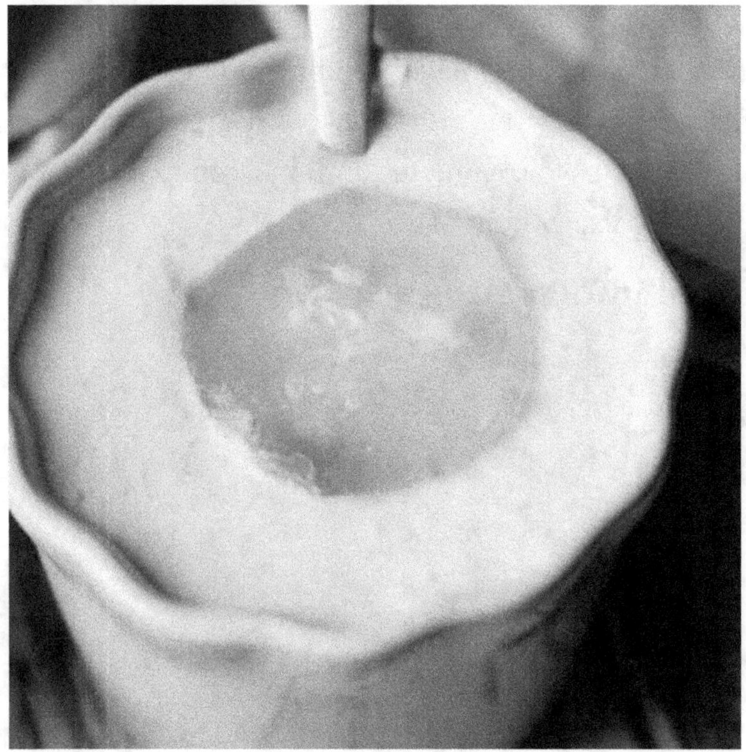

Prep time: 10 minutes
Cook time: 10 minutes
Servings: 10

Ingredients

- 1 cup of Greek yogurt
- 2 cups of grated and peeled cucumber
- 3 minced garlic clove
- 1 tbsp sesame paste (tahini)
- 1 lemon juice, squirt
- Salt, moderately to taste

Instructions

1. Mix all the aforementioned ingredients in a bowl and stir thoroughly.

2. What else? Consumption!

Nutritional information

Calories: 50

Protein: 2g

Net carbs: 1g

Fat: 12g

Ketogenic Desserts

Chocolate Cheesecake

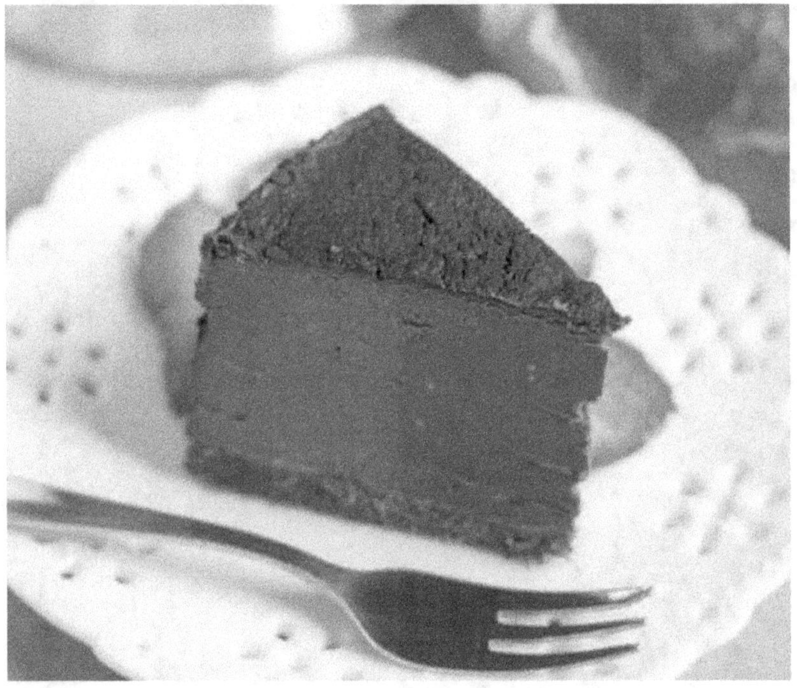

Prep time: 10 minutes
Cooking time: 35 minutes
Servings: 8

Ingredients

Crust

- 2 tbsp melted butter
- ¼ each almond and coconut flours
- 3 tbsp cocoa powder, unsweetened
- 2 tbsp keto sweetener

Filling

- 6 oz melted baking chocolate
- 1 tbsp vanilla extract
- ½ cup each heavy and sour creams
- ½ cup each stevia and monk fruit powders
- 1 cup vanilla extract
- 1/3 cup of cocoa powder, unsweetened
- 16 oz cream cheese
- 1 large egg and 2 yolks both at room temperature

Instructions

Crust

- First, spring form a pan with a parchment paper and then cut it accurately.
- Get a bowl to mix all the crust ingredients with the melted butter.

Filling

1. Blend sweeteners with cheese and the cocoa powder using an electric mixer.
2. Blend egg and the 2 egg yolks.
3. Blend the sour and heavy creams, extract and melted chocolate.
4. You can now spread the cheese mixture on the crust and use a spatula to smooth the top.
5. With about 2 cups of water, place the rack in the instant pot.
6. Place an extensive foil sling over the rack in order to reach both ends of the cooker.
7. In order to avoid condensate dripping, put the pan above the sling and slightly cover with foil.

8. Now, set the control of your cooker to maximum and leave it to cook for 20 minutes and then leave it to release naturally after the cooking for about 15 minutes.
9. Uncover the pot and place the cheesecake in a cooling rack using the sling.
10. Let it cool for 1 hour, then refrigerate it for some few hours and remove the pan sides.
11. For desired outcome, leave the cake in the refrigerator all night.
12. For it to be soft, target a room temperature.

Nutritional information

Calories: 413
Protein: 8g
Fat: 38g
Net carbs: 12g

Ricotta Lemon Cheesecake

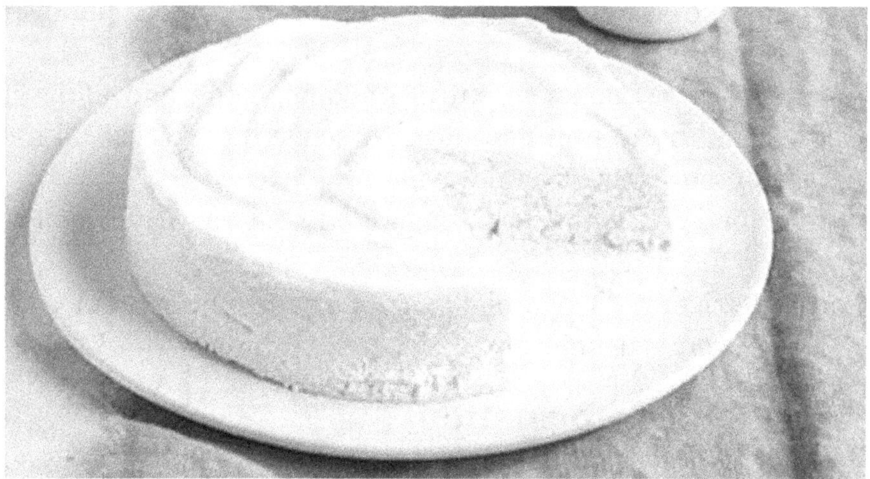

Prep time: 10 minutes
Cook time: 40 minutes
Servings: 6

Ingredients

- ¼ cup of trivia
- Zest and lemon juice from 1 lemon
- 1/3 cup cheese (Ricotta)
- 3 eggs
- 1 tsp extract from lemon
- 8 oz of cheese, creamy

Instructions

1. Use a stand mixer to mix all the ingredients save for the eggs.
2. Ensure the mixture is very smooth without lumps.
3. Lower the speed and then add the eggs and gently stir until they are fully blended.
4. Then, transfer it into a well-greased pan (6 inches spring-form, preferably) and cover it with a silicone lid.

5. At the bottom of the pot, place a trivet and pour in 2 cups of water. Then places the silicone covered pot over the trivet.
6. Set your cooker's control on high mode and allow it cook for 30 minutes and then leave it to release all the pressure in a natural way.
7. Now, gently mix the Truvia and sour cake and pour it on the cake.
8. Refrigerate it overnight or for about 7 hours and your dessert is deliciously ready!

Nutritional information

Calories: 181
Fat: 16g
Net carbs: 2g
Protein: 5g

Coconut Almond Cake

Preparation time: 10 minutes
Cook time: 40 minutes
Servings: 8

Ingredients

Wet ingredients

- 2 lightly whisked eggs
- ¼ cup of melted butter
- ½ cup of whipping cream, heavy one

Dry ingredients

- Apple pie spice and baking powder, 1 teaspoon each
- 1 cup of almond flour
- ½ cup of unsweetened coconut, shredded
- ½ cup of Truvia

Instructions

1. Start off by mixing all the dry ingredients together.
2. Then, start pouring in all the wet ingredients and mix appropriately until they all become blended.
3. Get a 6" pan cake and pour everything into it, then cover it with foil.
4. Fetch about 2 cups of water in the instant pot and a steamer rack over the pot.
5. It's time to set your instant pot control and guess what, it should just be a maximum of 40 minutes with 10 minutes release time!
6. With caution, bring out the pan and leave it to cool for 20 minutes.
7. Remove the cake into a clean plate and then, rub with almond and coconut oil. Ready to serve!

Nutritional information

Calories: 236
Net carbs: 5g
Protein: 6g
Fat: 23g
Saturated fat: 11g

Dark Chocolate Cake

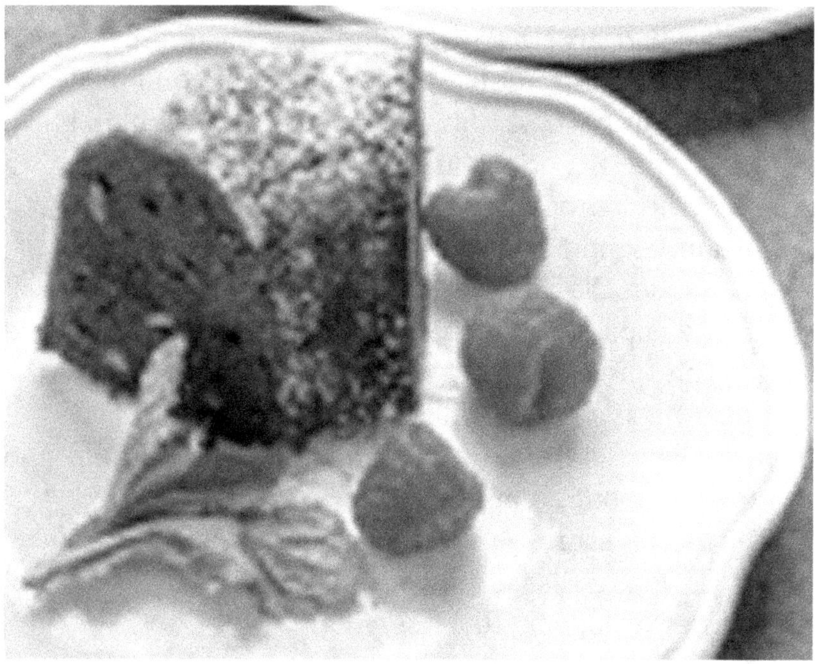

Prep time: 10 minutes
Cook time: 30 minutes
Servings: 6

Ingredients

- ¼ cup each finely chopped walnuts and unsweetened cocoa powder
- 1 cup of almond flour
- 3 large eggs
- ¼ of coconut oil
- 1 tsp baking powder
- 1/3 cup of whipping cream, heavy
- 2/3 cup Swerve

Instructions

1. With either an electric or hand mixer, carefully mix all the ingredients until they become well-combined and have a fluffy look. I'm pretty sure you wouldn't like dense cake. So, do the mixing very well.
2. Get a heat-proof pan that can perfectly fit into your instant pot and grease it.
3. Then, pour the mixed ingredients into the pan.
4. Pour 2 cups of water in the inner liner of your pot and get a steamer rack.
5. Cover the pot with a foil and place it on trivet.
6. With your cooker on high pressure, close the lid and cook for about 20 minutes.
7. Let the pressure be manually released for 10 minutes before you release the remnants.
8. The next step, ooh, that's serving!

Nutritional information

Calories: 301
Net carbs: 7g
Protein: 8g
Fat: 28g

Almond Carrot cake

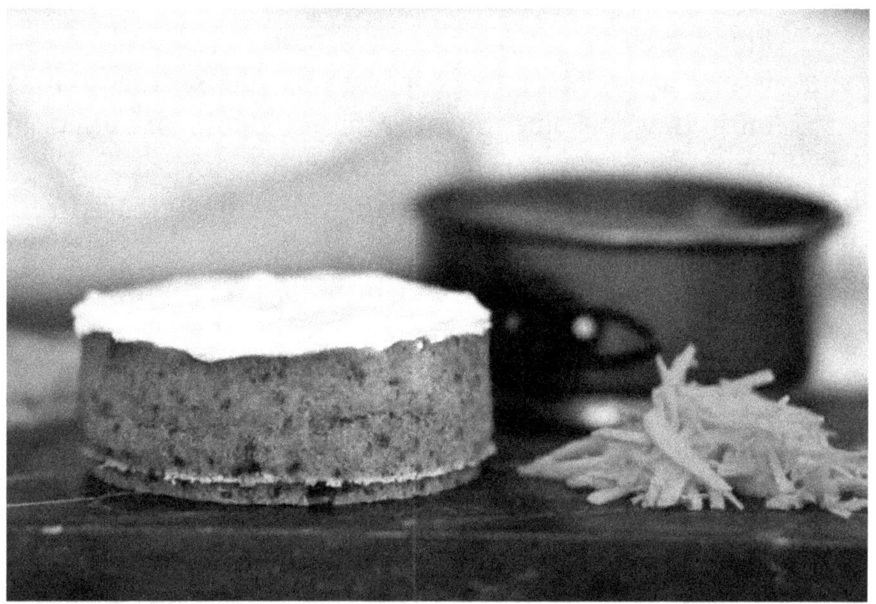

Preparation time: 10 minutes

Cook time: 50 minutes

Servings: 8

Ingredients

- 3 large eggs
- 1 tsp baking powder
- ¼ cup of coconut oil
- ½ cup each finely chopped walnuts and heavy whipping cream, half cup each
- 1 cup of shredded carrots
- 1 ½ tsp of apple pie spice
- 1 cup of almond flour
- 2/3 cup swerve

Instructions

1. Finely grease your 6 inches cake pan.
2. Use a hand-mixer to properly mix all the ingredients until they become fluffy. Almond flours are fond of being dense if not properly mixed.
3. Pour everything into the pan you earlier greased and cover it with foil.
4. Now, fetch 2 cups of water into the inner liner of your pot and gently place the pan on trivet.
5. Hit the 'cake' button on your cooker and allow 40 minutes cooking. However, if there's no cake button on your cooker, bother less! Just set the time of the device to 40 minutes and you'll get the same result.
6. After that, let the pressure release manually for 10 minutes before you release the other pressure by yourself.
7. After cooling, you may put icing or just enjoy it as it is!

Nutritional information

Calories: 268
Protein: 6g
Net carbs: 5g
Fat: 25g

Coconut Panda Custard

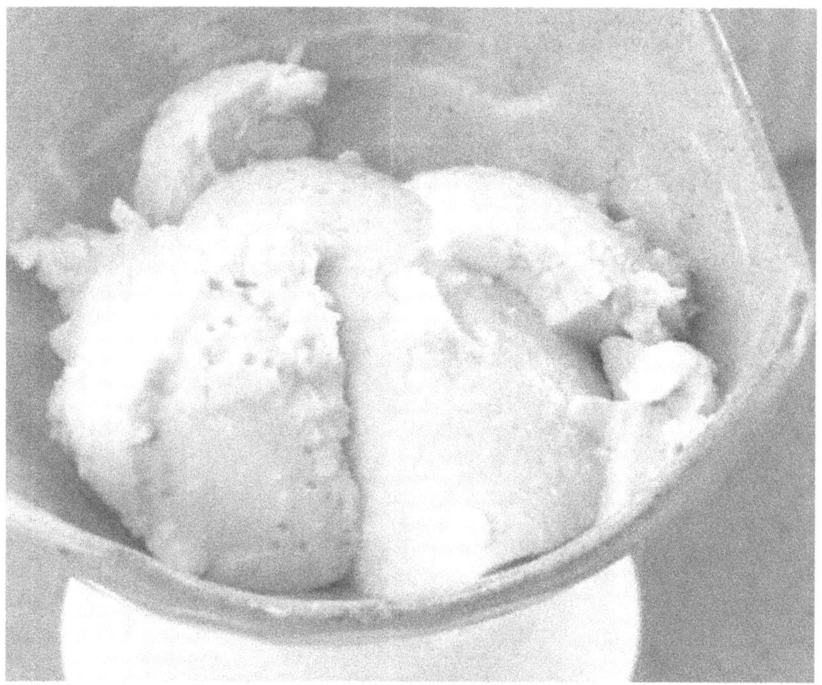

Prep time: 5 minutes
Cook time: 30 minutes
Servings: 4

Ingredients

- 3 large eggs
- 4 drops of panda extract
- 1 cup of unsweetened coconut milk
- 1/3 Truvia blend

Instructions

1. Blend all the ingredients together.
2. Pour the blended ingredients into a 6-inch heat-proof plate, then use foil to cover it.

3. Pour 2 cups of water into the inner liner of your instant pot and place the trivet on the liner and carefully drop the plate in the trivet.
4. Set the control of your pot to maximum and allow 30 minutes cooking.
5. Let it naturally release pressure for some minutes.
6. Now, place it in your refrigerator and patiently wait for this yummy dessert to be set!

Nutritional information

Calories: 174
Net carbs: 4g
Protein: 6g
Fat: 14g

Chocolate Mousse

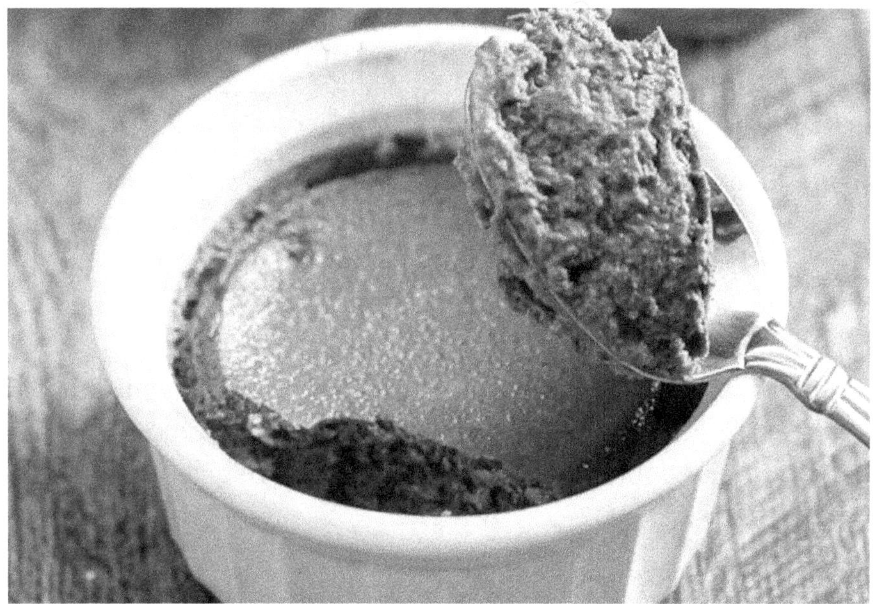

Prep time: 10 minutes
Cook time: 20 minutes
Servings: 5

Ingredients

- ¼ cup each water and cacao
- 4 egg yolks
- ½ cup each swerve and almond milk
- 1 cup of whipping cream
- Sea salt, a dash
- ½ tbsp vanilla

Instructions

1. Put the egg yolks into a bowl and stir thoroughly.
2. Get a sauce pan to mix the water, cacao and swerve. Stir continuously until everything becomes blended.

3. Now, add the almond milk and cream to the pan and allow it to heat up without boiling.
4. Add in the vanilla and salt and mix thoroughly.
5. Add 1 tablespoonful of chocolate mixture into the yolks and stir to rightly combine.
6. Transfer the mixtures into a jar.
7. Add about 2 cups of water into the liner of your pot and a trivet above it and conspicuously place the jar on the trivet.
8. Cover it and allow 6 minutes of cooking.
9. After that, release and take off the jars. Ideally, they'll be hot, so you need something to remove them.
10. After cooling on the counter, then refrigerate it for 6 hours.

Nutritional information

Calories: 246
Net carbs: 2g
Protein: 6g
Fat: 15g